The Best Constipation Remedies

"Here are proven natural, constipation remedies that you need to give you a clean mind and to help you start a new life."

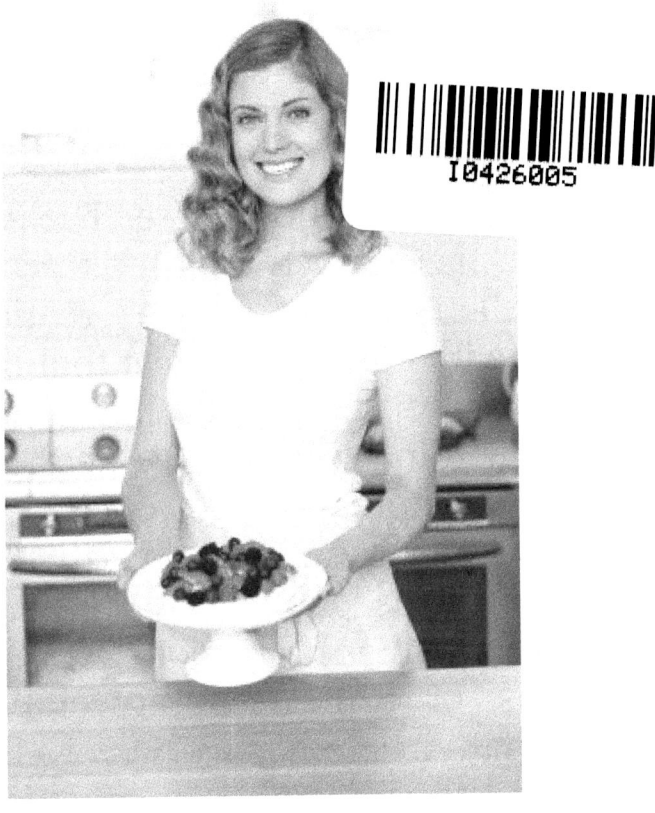

By Rudy S Silva, Natural Nutritionist

The Best Constipation Remedies © 2012 (updated 2014) by Rudy S Silva

ISBN-13: 978-1492958505
ISBN-10: 1492958506

Disclaimer and Terms of Use: The Author and Publisher has strived to be as accurate and complete as possible in the creation of this book, notwithstanding the fact that he does not warrant or represent at any time that the contents within are accurate due to the rapidly changing nature of research. While all attempts have been made to verify information provided in this publication, the Author and Publisher assumes no responsibility for errors, omissions, or contrary interpretation of the subject matter herein. Any perceived slights of specific persons, peoples, or organizations are unintentional.

The information in this article is not intended as medical advice, to diagnose, treat, cure or prevent any disease. It is information provided for your education and knowledge and not to take the place of going to the doctor for medical treatment and advice. The U.S. FDA has not approved these products listed here. Consult your doctor when using new remedies or techniques when dealing with various illness or symptoms. The information in this book is intended for educational and informational purposes only. In using this knowledge, you do at your own risk.

First Printing, 2012 Printed in the United States of America

Table of Contents

1: Introduction to Constipation

Seventy percent or more of the population struggles with constipation. Some believe the number is even higher, 80-90%. The market for laxatives is now approaching 1 billion or more each year. It appears that constipation is an issue that most of us have to deal with at one time or the other. Using natural means to clear constipation is what this book is all about.

The first question that a nutritionist or any other health practitioner should ask you on your first visit is, "how many bowel movements do you have each day or each week?"

Your Doctor and Constipation

If you visit a doctor, your colon is the last area they discuss with you. Or, this might be an area they may never discuss with you at all.

In his article, The Bowel is an Ecosystem, in Healthy & Natural Journal, April 1997, Majid

Ali, M.D. recounts,

"When I returned to the clinical practice of environmental and nutritional medicine after years of pathology work, I began carefully testing the assertions of nutritionists, naturopaths and clinical ecologist who claimed that various types of colitis [a deterioration of your colon wall could be reversed with optimal nutritional and ecologic approaches. To my great surprise, I found that such professionals, who are usually spurned by drug doctors, were right after all. My patients responded well to the unscientific therapies vehemently rejected by my colleagues in drug medicine."

The Foundation of Colon Health

There are many excellent books available on colon health and constipation; you should also look into them. This book has many quotes from these books. The authors of these books have put down the foundation for the knowledge we have about how your colon works and how to keep it healthy.

By concentrating on eliminating constipation and preserving colon health, you have taken a major step in preventing body conditions that can shorten your life or make your senior years a miserable time.

The Importance of Colon Health

Your colon is one of the most important organs that you should concentrate on keeping healthy. This will help you   avert many unnecessary illnesses and sufferings.

Heart attacks, cancers, senility, pathogenic organisms cause most deaths in the US and throughout the world. There are fewer deaths related to natural causes or old age.

Your colon provides nutrients and water to all parts of the body. So, when a specific organ is losing function, it is important to see what part colon toxins have played in this deterioration.

If your colon is toxic, your blood will also be toxic. If your colon is toxic, these toxins will gradually reach all parts of the body through the blood and lymph liquid. The result is the body and various organs affected will become less efficient. Overtime this decreased efficiency will cause the body will become diseased.

By not eating clean food and without good colon health, you will be a victim of your own poisoning. It was estimated that of all the people who died of cancer – colon, lung, prostate, and breast – in 1999 sixteen percent were attributed to colon cancer. But, how many of these other cancers originated in your colon? We do know that colon cancer is the second leading cause of deaths in the United States.

It is the nutritionist's job to tell you what foods, nutrients, and supplements you need to prevent and to overcome specific illnesses.

Why People Die so Young

Why is it that so many people are dying of various diseases at such an early age – at forty, at fifty, at sixty, even 30, or younger? They die of heart diseases, blood diseases, cancers, autoimmune diseases, and the list goes on. It has been known for a longtime why diseases occur and what you can do to prevent them.

But the public is not willing to undertake the steps necessary to stop these illnesses. These death producing illnesses are a result of lifestyle - the foods we eat, the water we drink, the air pollution we breathe, the thoughts we think, the toxins we are exposed to at work, and the cleaning products we use at home.

It takes disciple to change behavior, thought, and lifestyle, which are good for health. This is what is necessary to reduce or eliminate illness. This is what is necessary to bring on a feeling of well-being way into your old age – at 80, at 90, at 100, and way beyond that. With the new anti-aging nutrients and supplements on the market, some people are living well over a 100 years, provided they follow a good lifestyle.

How many people are willing to take on this rigorous challenge now at age 20, even younger or older? Most young people are not thinking about their health, since at this age their body has not weakened enough to produce enough body pain. They have a body that can bounce back from misuse and from a poor lifestyle. But, with every day that passes, their capacity to bounce back changes by a small unnoticeable amount. Then, like a rubber band that loses it spring, this young person, now older, begins to feel the detrimental effects of the lifestyle they have been living.

This book will help you clear and eliminate constipation. It gives you information about your colon, so you can decide how to keep it clean and healthy.

It takes some work to do it. But you are going to be eating, thinking, and living, so why not do it right and let go of the unhealthy habits. It is your choice. Now, take the right path.

Do It One Step at A Time

As Robert Gray says in his book, your colon Health Handbook, 1980-2000,

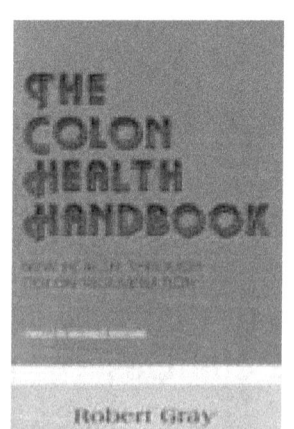

"Nearly every man, women, child in modern society today is constipated. Yes constipated whether they know it or not. Yes, constipated even though the bowels might move regularly every day. Yes, even people with chronic diarrhea suffer from one form of constipation."

So, you cannot avoid having to deal with the symptoms of constipation or with constipation itself. If you do then, you place yourself at risk to come down with illness after illness, as you get older.

This book provides you with time-tested remedies that are all natural - foods, minerals, vitamins, and various nutrients.

Consult your doctor when using new remedies or techniques when dealing with constipation or associated symptoms. Be especially alert when you notice blood in your stools, have a different color stool, have a pencil like stool, have stomach or abdominal pain, have a change in bowel frequency, or have been constipated for 2-3 weeks or more. Under these conditions consult your doctor.

Constipation can be a symptom of more serious illnesses such as diverticulosis, colon cancer, colitis, and others. The information provided here is for educational use and is not a prescription for any illness, discomfort, or disease. It is information for your knowledge and not to take the place of going to your doctor for medical treatment and advice.

2: Types of Constipation You Might Have

Types of Constipation

There are two types of constipation, organic and functional.

Organic constipation is a result of some physical change, obstruction, or distortion in your colon. This type of constipation needs immediate attention from a doctor. We do not cover constipation that occurs for these reasons.

Functional constipation is a result of not following a proper diet, drinking the proper liquids, having good emotional health, and not having the proper lifestyle that promotes good movement of digested foods through your intestines and colon.

Even though there are many conditions, symptoms and definitions describing constipation, constipation simple is a condition where the fecal matter going through your colon remains there too long, before moving out of your rectum.

Constipation is a symptom that tells you your colon is not working properly, or you have some underlying gastrointestinal disease you are not aware of.

Constipation is a warning your diet and lifestyle can be leading to some illness or disease in the future. It is a symptom that many people ignore, or a symptom that many people try to eliminate by using dangerous drugstore laxatives.

Laxatives are probable the worst product you can use, when you have constipation. They can become habit-forming, if used too long and have some nasty side effects. They have a tendency to create the problem you are trying to relieve – constipation.

In the following chapters, you will get some of the best natural remedies that have been documented to work for constipation. It is important to use only natural remedies for constipation, so you don't continue to upset the natural balance and function of your colon.

As you begin to apply some of these remedies, keep in mind that one particular remedy does not work for everyone. You may have to make some changes to some of these remedies, such as increasing dosage, adding other remedies, or trying different substances.

The remedies you choose to use will depend on specific herbs, foods, or nutrients you have, you can buy locally, you can buy on the Internet, or can afford.

Experimenting is part of how you find out what is best for you.
Keep in mind that all remedies listed here should be used only for a short time, one week and not longer than 4 weeks. After 4 weeks, use a different remedy. They should only be used for the time needed to clear your constipation. Sometimes this might just be three or six times.

There are some herbal combinations, you can use longer. These combinations can improve the health of your colon and get your bowels moving.

Health Tip: After you clear your constipation, you need to learn what it takes to create a healthy colon, so your constipation doesn't come back. This is the most important part of dealing with your constipation.

When fecal matter remains in your colon for days, your colon becomes toxic and spreads this toxicity into every part of your body.

In the bloodstream, these toxins interfere with the delivery of oxygen to your cells and tissues.

If you have to strain and squeeze to have a bowel movement, you can damage the tissues in the lower part of your colon and the blood vessels in your legs.

In the Past

Over 90 years ago or more, doctors knew about the importance of a clean colon. In 1908, Eli Metchnifoff, director of the Pasteur Institute, was awarded the Nobel Prize for Medicine. His research showed that pathogenic colon bacteria, bad bacteria (To be covered in a later chapter) produced toxic secretions and by products, which acted as slow poisoning of the entire body.

Metchnifoff believed that toxic matter coming from your colon was responsible for every degenerating disease. His belief was so strong that he suggested that man's life span was certainly cut in half, when his colon was neglected and allowed to have excessive toxic producing bacteria.

In 1931 Dr. Joseph H. Greer, was telling his patients what to do to end constipation and how to prevent it. Today, nutritionists and other health practitioners are telling their clients the same thing.

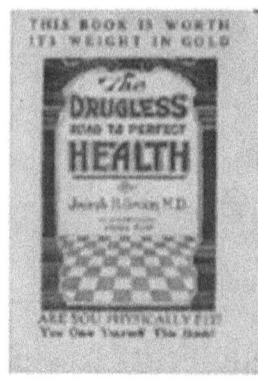

In his small book, The Drugless Road to Perfect Health, 1931, Joseph H. Greer, M.D. reminded his patients, "You must have 'roughage' to make the bowels move freely. Concentrated food (processed foods) and constipation go hand in hand, (and) then pills (laxatives) are used. More constipation and more pills, it is a vicious circle with bad results. Don't be afraid of cracked wheat, cornmeal, cut oats, raw cabbage, onions and celery. They are far better than refined flour and the package foods that flood the market. They may save some labor in the kitchen, but they produce constipation."

In 1981, Dr. Jensen in his book, Tissue Cleansing Through

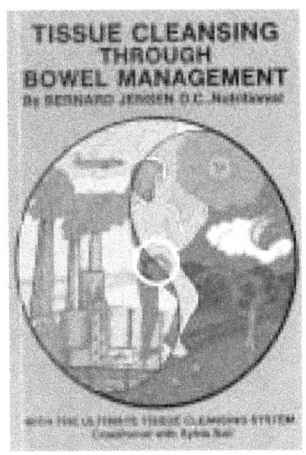

Bowel Management, Dr. Jensen said, "I believe that when the bowel is under active, toxic wastes are more likely to be absorbed through the bowel wall and into the bloodstream from which they become deposited in the tissues... As toxins accumulate in the tissues, increasing degrees of cell destruction take place...proper function is slowed in all body tissues in which toxins have settled.

When anyone has reached the degenerative disease stage, it is a sign that toxic settlements have taken the body over."

Today, it is well accepted by nutritionists, Naturopathic doctors, and other alternative medicine practitioners that constipation is a signal that cannot be ignored and your colon function must be kept efficient and well-functioning.

Constipation is a symptom you cannot ignore – even if it occurs only occasionally, because it leads to slow poisoning of your entire body.

Many doctors, for a longtime, have refused to believe that constipation can cause other parts of the body to become weaken and become unable to perform their function. You will still find Internet articles, anatomy books, and health books suggesting that for some people bowel movements in three days or more can be normal.

Some doctors don't want to admit that when your fecal matter stays in your colon for more than 36 hours, you may have constipation.

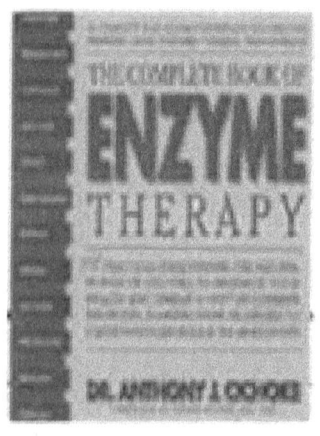

In his book, The Complete book of Enzyme Therapy, 1999, Dr. Anthony J. Cichoke, says that "The frequency of bowel movements depends on your physical make-up and physical and dietary habits. Most people have one movement every twenty-four hours, but some individuals have a movement every thirty-six or forty-eight hours (or at even greater intervals) and do not suffer from constipation. There is nothing to worry about if you have only occasional minor discomfort or irregularity."

But then Dr. Cichoke continues,

"Unless constipation is the result of an organic disease, it is rarely serious in itself, but it can lead to diverticulitis and diverticulosis. Toxic build-up in your colon can lead to colon cancer."

Since constipation does not result in immediate ill symptoms, many doctors believe that constipation is not a problem. Doctors wait until there is a degradation of your health. This is something they can measure and see. By this time, it is difficult to relate the disease back to a toxic colon or to where it originated.

This results in the use of drugs or surgery to remove the ill condition and meanwhile, the cause of the illness is not taken care of. Doctors will continue to prescribe drugs, thinking that the cause has been addressed.

You do not have to wait for a disease to take hold of your body, so doctors can prescribe you drugs. Take responsibility for your health and don't let constipation become a reoccurring condition.

In her booklet, Natural Relief from

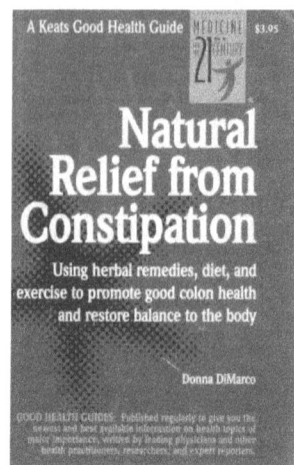

A Keats Good Health Guide MEDICINE $3.95

Natural Relief from Constipation

Using herbal remedies, diet, and exercise to promote good colon health and restore balance to the body

Donna DiMarco

Constipation, 1999, Donna Di Marco, a Nutritional Counselor, says, "Nearly twenty years ago, the prestigious medical journal, the Lancet, reported that women who have two or fewer bowel movements each week have four times the risk of breast disease (benign or malignant) as women who have one or more bowel movements each day."

When you have constipation, take it as a serious problem you need to take off. If you do, then you will add many happy years to your life.

Don't fall for the opinion of some in the health industry that say, if you don't have a bowel movement every day this is OK. It is not all right, and it is not OK.

If you are eating 3 meals a day and have only one bowel movement each day, your meals are backing up in your colon. They are staying longer in your colon than they should.

In Tom Monte's book, The Complete Guide to

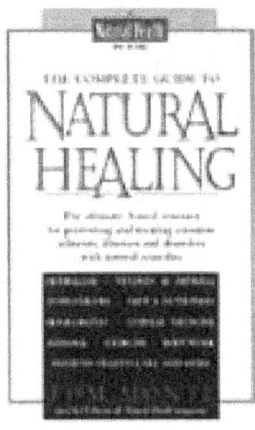

Natural Healing, 1997, he says, "Intestinal health is fundamental to the overall good health of the body. Ideally, people should have an adequate bowel movement once a day, but years on the highly refined Western diet may have made that goal impossible for many. In that case, ample and regular bowel movements every other day should be the norm."

Health Alert: If you have a long-standing problem with constipation or severe constipation, you should see your doctor for advice.

3: Are You Really Constipated?

Definition of Constipation

Elimination of waste products that come from your stomach, small intestines, and colon are part of your digestive process. When waste matter or fecal matter slows down or stops moving in your colon, the entire digestive process is affected. Your health depends on having good digestion.

Constipation sometimes referred to as irregularity, can be defined in many ways. Some people believe that constipation is when you don't have more than three bowel movements each week. Others believe that less than one bowel movement each day is constipation.

You might believe that constipation is when you have a hard time in the bathroom straining and puffing to have a bowel movement.

Here is another definition of constipation,

Fecal matter that moves slowly or stops, which allows toxic chemicals to pass through your colon walls and into your bloodstream is constipation.

There are over 100s of different toxic chemicals that exist in your colon. Some come from undigested protein, by-products of digestion, bacteria fermentation, additives from processed foods, which decay in your colon, and from food that has existed in your colon for years. Some of these toxins are more harmful than others, so it is critical that these poisons do not get into your bloodstream.

In her article, The Road to Reversing MCS/EI is Paved With Good Intestines, The Townsend Letter for Doctors – January 2000, Dr. Gloria Gilbere states,

"Intestinal poisoning not manifesting immediate visible effects appear in disorders such as MCS, fibromyalgia, chronic fatigue, lupus, and arthritis, to mention a few. Eventually, the chemicals produced by putrefaction are so poisonous they irritate the delicate lining of the large intestine and destroy the protective barrier keeping out the invading toxins. Damage from the chemical toxins is so destructive your colon walls become leaky and allow penetration through the damaged barrier into the lymphatic and circulatory systems, especially through the hepatic portal vein."

For fecal matter to slow down in your colon, as if some blockage was present, requires certain colon activities or processes to malfunction. It requires certain mental, emotional, and unhealthy conditions to exist, which affect the proper function of your colon.

Fecal Matter Transit Time

The time fecal matter stays in your colon before toxins start to stream into your blood will vary. But, there is a typical transit time for food to travel from your mouth and out of your anus. This transit time is around 16 – 22 hours. This time is considered normal and times outside this period are something to work on, by changing your eating habits.

Yes, it is true that certain people have faster or slower transit times than others. The question to ask of those people, whose transient time is slow, 2-3 day, is why is it slow? The response should not be that this is normal because that's just the way their colon works.

What are the main conditions that affect transient time?

- Colon wall muscles have become weak and un-toned
- Colon wall nerves have been damaged through an excess use of laxatives
- The amount of food you have eaten
- The amount of water you drink during the day
- The type of food you have eaten
- The way you have chewed your food
- Your emotional condition
- A deficiency in specific minerals

These are a few conditions that affect your colon transient time and there are others, which are discussed in another chapter.

The longer fecal matter stays in your colon, the more it decomposes, decays, and putrefies.

This is the condition that causes toxic matter to move into your blood and to weaken and destroy your colon wall cells and tissue.

Number of Bowel Movements

If you have one, two or more bowel movements a day, you may still be constipated. If you sit on the toilet and have to stay there over 5- 10 minutes pushing, straining, or paining to have a bowel movement, then you are constipated. Straining to have a bowel movement, overtime, leads to hemorrhoids, varicose veins, or fissures.

If you eat three meals a day, then you should have three bowel movements each day. The first bowel movement should take place in the morning, when you wake up or soon after you have had breakfast. Typical you should experience the urge for a bowel movement 20-30 minutes after you eat. The other bowel movements should be during the day and just before bedtime.

In her book, Healthy Digestion the Natural way, 2000, D. Lindsey Berkson defines constipation as,

"A healthy person should have at least one

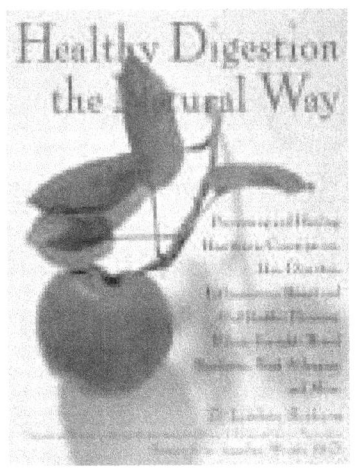

bowel movement a day. Medical textbooks state that individual variation goes from several times a day to several times a week. However, having worked with people for many years on improving their health, I would define constipation as not having one to several daily bowel movements, or having too long an intestinal-transit time."

If you eat three meals a day and only have one or two bowel movements, then the second and third meal are backing up in your colon and staying there too long.

When your fecal matter stays too long in your colon, water is pulled out of the fecal matter and reabsorbed through your colon wall. This makes the fecal matter stiff and hard. Your colon will now have a hard time moving this hard fecal matter through its sections and out the rectum.

Definition of Constipation Expanded

So, Constipation is when:

- It takes more than 18-25 hours for food to travel from your mouth to your anus
- Slow moving fecal matter in your colon allows time for toxins to move into your bloodstream.
- You develop hemorrhoids, fissures, diverticulosis, or varicose veins
- You eat three times a day and only have one bowel movement
- You strain and push to have a bowel movement
- Your stools are hard and dry

Doctors and Constipation

Of course, doctors do not consider constipation a serious medical issue, unless it becomes persistent, or it starts to occur frequently for no known reason.

So doctors have a different definition of constipation.

When a person complains about constipation,

many doctors do not know what causes it or how to treat it. Especially, if they cannot make direct measurements that indicate the body is malfunctioning, or they cannot see any unnatural physical condition, using various scanners. So they will normally prescribe a laxative. Or, they may tell you, if your bowel movements have been occurring every three days for years, then this is normal.

A main concern you should have about constipation is whether toxins are getting into your body – autointoxication. Over a long period of time autointoxication creates illness and irreversible organ damage. This is something a doctor will not tell you about constipation. Most doctors don't subscribe to the idea that your colon spreads toxins into your body, which are responsible for serious illnesses.

When your colon starts spreading toxins into your bloodstream, these toxins are transported to everybody cell, body joint and to all body organs. To prevent this from happenings, you need to eliminate constipation and detoxify your colon.

Recently, Loree Taylor Jordan, Colonic

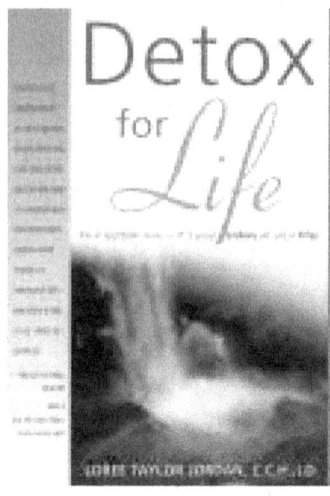 Therapist, wrote in her book Detox for Life, 2002, that, "If you ask the average physician about autointoxication, trust me, s/he will most likely downplay your concerns. The average doctor in general does not have any concept of how to detoxify the body and most certainly does not relate it to disease control. Of course, there are also any doctors who do support detoxification. My intent is not to criticize the medical profession. It provides a great service, but many practitioners are just not trained to new concepts in the field of nutrition and disease prevention through detoxification."

Occasional Constipation

Doctors will tell you that an occasional bout with constipation is nothing to worry about. If you don't have a bowel movement every day, this is also nothing to worry about. Some doctors don't want to admit that when your fecal matter stays in your colon for more than 36 hours, you may have a constipation problem.

They consider constipation normal, if you have a bowel movement from three times each day to one time a week. You may have a bowel movement once in three days, and doctors will consider this normal.

How many of us have constipation occasionally. What does occasionally mean? Does it mean once a week, once a month, or once a year? And, why are drug store laxatives the most often purchased drug or supplement? The laxative market is approaching a billion dollar industry. Is this a sign that all of us are constipated occasionally?

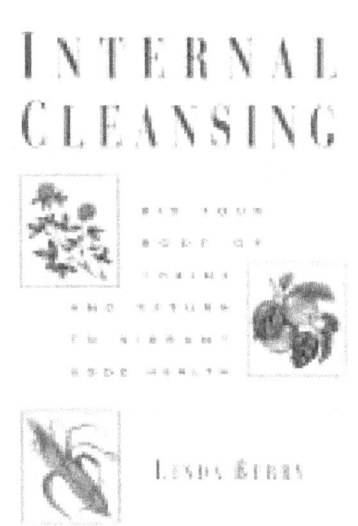

In her book, Internal Cleansing, 1997, Linda Berry recalls, "Recently, two patients came to my office suffering with serious constipation. One was having, at best five bowel movements each week. The other said he had eliminated only once every four days since he was a small boy. Perhaps your medical doctor – like that of the first patient – has told you that this level of excretion is okay.

Her doctor's perspective was that some people just have fewer bowel movements than others. That is true, but what he neglected to tell her is that those who have fewer bowel movements are harboring a breeding ground for disease and death."

Constipation is a Serious Problem

Most people have some form constipation and they don't know how important it is not to have it.

When you do become constipated, you try to identify why this has occurred. Is it because you have started taking medical drugs, changed your diet, not eating enough fiber, eating too many processed foods, or going through some emotional issue?

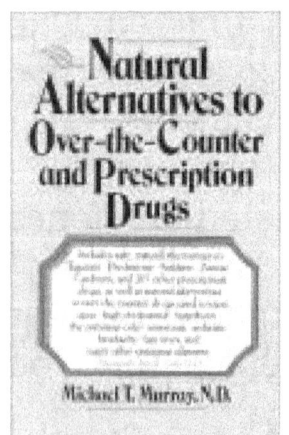

In, Natural Alternatives to Over-the-Counter and Prescription Drugs, 1994, Michael T. Murray, N.D. says, "Since the frequency of defecation and the consistency and volume of stools vary so greatly from individual to individual, it is difficult to determine what is normal.

Nonetheless, most nutritionally oriented physicians consider two to three bowel movements each day as ideal. This is the number that is typically found in healthy people eating a high-fiber diet and getting adequate exercise."

Health Alert: If you experience a change in bowel movement frequency that is unexplainable and persistent, consider this a warning and see your doctor. Sudden changes in bowel movement frequency, which last for some time, can be a symptom of some other underlying disease.

Constipation is a signal you are not treating your body with right food, thought, and activity. It is an opportunity for you to make changes so you will not create a serious illness.

Constipation Defined More
Another definition of constipation is:

Fecal matter that is stagnant and backs up in your colon

This means that if you have a bowel movement and not all the fecal matter, which is in your colon, comes out, then this is constipation.

If not all the fecal matter comes out and some of it remains in your colon, then this is considered stagnant fecal matter. If this fecal matter remains, as it does in many individuals and continues to build up on your colon walls overtime, then this is considered constipation.

It is constipation, since it is stagnant fecal matter that is not coming out during a bowel movement. This build-up of fecal matter on your colon wall is called "Mucoid Plaque," since it is a layer of fecal matter and mucus.

In his pamphlet, Your Colon Health Handbook, 1980-2000, Robert Gray points out two types of constipation.

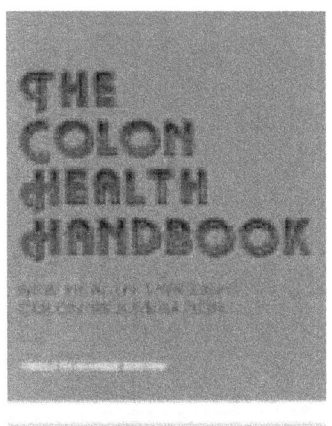

"There are two types of constipation. One type is present when the feces that pass from the body are overly packed together. Another type of constipation is present when old, hardened feces stick to the walls of your colon and do not pass out with the regular bowel movements. Both types of constipation are so common among the members of modern society today that scarcely anybody recognizes them as being unnatural. As we shall see, constipated bowel movements are generally looked upon as normal stools. And few people have any inkling as to how much old, hardened feces are chronically present within their bodies."

Here are some of the signs you are constipated:

- Abdomen pain
- Acne
- Appetite loss

- Asthma
- Bad breathe
- Coated tongue
- Epilepsy
- Fever
- Headaches
- Hypertension
- Mental dullness
- Mucus coated tongue
- Nausea
- No bowel movements during the day
- Pain in the lower legs
- Skin disorders
- Stomach heaviness
- Straining to have a bowel movement
- Tiredness

4: How Drugstore Laxatives can ruin Your Colon

Laxatives

A laxative is defined as,

A substance that is used to promote a bowel movement, when you are constipated

Laxatives work by starting and stimulating peristaltic action. Peristaltic action is a wave-like movement that occurs throughout your gastrointestinal tract – esophagus, stomach, small intestine, and colon. This action helps move food into your stomach, through your intestines, through your colon, and out of your rectum.

There are drugstore products, natural occurring foods, herbal substances, and homeopathic liquids that have laxative effects. If possible, you should avoid drugstore laxatives or any other form of drugs to clear constipation.

All my recommendations are for using natural foods, minerals, or herbal products. And, some of these natural methods should only be used for the time it takes to clear your constipation.

Health Alert: You should use drug store or drug laxatives only under Doctor's recommendations.

There are no safe drugstore laxatives. These laxatives are habit- forming and work by desensitizing your colon. Their use can,

- irritate nerves and muscles along the intestinal lining
- interfere with digestion and adsorption
- cause cramps
- deplete fluids
- create physical internal problems.

Laxatives can enlarge and seriously damage your colon when used for a long time. Eventually, after continual use, you will not be able to have a bowel movement, without using them.

Health Alert: Never use a laxative, Drugstore or Natural, when you have acute abdominal pain, especially if the pain is on the lower right-hand side, where the appendix is located. See your doctor right away.

Using Laxatives for the wrong reason can be life threatening.

What Drugstore Laxative Do

If you are tempted to use drugstore laxatives remember that,

Laxatives bought in drugstores are of questionable safety.

Because of the action these laxatives have on the small intestine and colon, doctors and other health practitioners recommend their limited. These laxatives have chemical side effects that affect your health. They produce an active force that can damage nerves that control the muscles in your colon walls. In addition, they,

- desensitize your colon so your natural peristaltic action is reduced
- become habit-forming
- rush food through your intestines, so it

does not digest and absorb nutrients or minerals properly

- kill friendly bacteria, unless they are fiber foods
- Contain preservatives, coloring, and other additives that are unhealthy.
- remove excessive fluids and electrolytes

Health Alert: If you use drugstore laxative, use them for just the time needed to clear your constipation. Then, starting looking at what it takes to stop your constipation from occurring.

Health Tip: When you have constipation, always start with the gentlest and safest laxative.

Five Basic Types of Drugstore Laxatives

There are five basic types of drugstore laxatives you should be aware of. Some of these laxatives are combinations of these five types, which are designed to create an effective constipation product. In making this combination, they create a product that is more dangerous to your health.

1. Bulk Forming Laxatives – clears constipation in 1-3 days

2. Stool Softening Laxatives – Emollients – works in 1-4 days

3. Lubricant Laxatives – works in 5- 9 hours

4. Osmotic or Saline Chemical Laxatives – works 1- 3 hours

5. Stimulant Laxatives – works in 6 – 24 hours

If you are going to use any of these laxatives keep in mind they will work faster when you take them on an empty stomach.

Bulk Forming Laxatives

Bulking laxatives are the safest laxative to use and can be use longer than other types of laxatives. These laxatives contain fiber or fiber like products. However, it is best to get your fiber from food, since food has a balance of all nutrients your body needs.

These laxatives work by making your stools larger and heavier and help attract and trap water into their fiber structure. This stimulates your colon to have a bowel movement. Using laxatives that contain fiber is a natural way to stimulate your colon into action. Bulking products or food can be used for mild cases of constipation.

Use them with plenty of water, so the bulking material does not expand in your throat or cause a backup in your colon. Using an excess of bulking products daily, can cause the problem you are trying to eliminate - constipation.

Natural bulking agents are pectin, guar, agar, and psyllium seed. Some semi-synthetic bulking agents that you want to avoid are methylcellulose or carboxy-methyl cellulose.

Drug Store Laxatives

Some bulk forming laxatives you will find in the drugstore are:

- Citrucel – contains methylcellulose (not recommended)

- Fiberall – contains psyllium seeds

- Fibercon – contains Calcium Polycarbophil (not recommended) Hydrocil – contains psyllium seeds
- Metamucil – contains psyllium husks
- Perdiem Fiber – contains senna
- Ultrafiber – contains psyllium seeds and prunes

Health Alert: Some bulk forming laxatives contain excess sugar and sodium. Read the label for these ingredients, if you have high blood pressure or are diabetic.

If you are pregnant, using bulk forming laxatives may be the safest way to relieve your constipation, but look for natural fiber food products. These natural products are discussed in other chapters.

Avoid using any non-bulking laxatives, since the chemicals, they contain can get into the fetus when breast- feeding.

Stool Softener Laxatives – Emollients

Stool softeners and emollients work by absorbing water into the fecal matter. This makes the fecal matter softer, so it can pass easier through your colon and out the rectum. Two of the chemicals used in stool softener laxatives are

- docusate sodium

- docusate calcium.

Don't use these types of laxatives since they have chemicals that can produce side effects. Docusate sodium has been found to increase the toxicity of drugs, when taken at the same time. In addition, they affect liver function.

You can find some of these laxatives at your local drugstore under the names,

- Colace – contains docusate sodium

- Dialose – contains docusate sodium

- Surfak – contains docusate calcium

Other products that contain docusate sodium and docusate calcium are:

- Senokot-S, Correctol 50 plus

- Fleet Stool Softener,

- Phillips Liquid-Gel

Health Alert: Avoid using docusate with mineral oil, since these increases the chances of absorbing some mineral oil into the body. Mineral oil in your body tissues can form tumors.

Pregnant women should avoid using Stool softeners and emollients laxatives.

Lubricant Stool Softeners

Lubricants stimulate a bowel movement by coating your colon walls and your fecal matter. These lubricants also help keep water in the fecal matter, preventing them from becoming hard and difficult to pass through your colon and rectum. One such lubricant is mineral oil – (not recommended).

Health Alert: Avoid laxatives that contain mineral oils. These oils can cause a pneumonia that is difficult to clear. They interfere with intestinal absorption of nutrients, and fat-soluble vitamins, like vitamin A. These lubricants collect in the lymph nodes when used often.

Mineral oil is not a food. It coats food and prevents it from being digested and prevents absorption of vitamins and nutrients. Dale Alexander, author of Arthritis Common Sense, 1981, reminds us that, "Crude mineral oil was discovered, by Indians, on top of stagnant

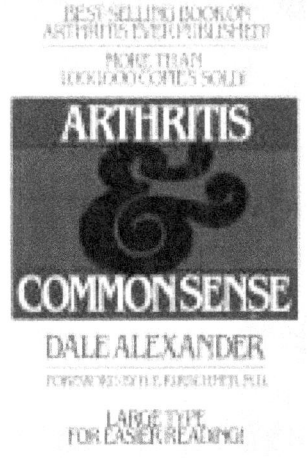

water in the oil fields. Today, mineral oil is refined into pure from petroleum. Refineries could not sell mineral oil for automobile use, so their representatives educated people to pour it into their bodies. Just the way mineral oil does not pass qualifications for a car carburetor. It forms puddles of useless oil in your intestinal loops."

Mineral oil passes from the mouth, all the way through your colon, and out the rectum without being absorbed. However, it sometimes passes through the intestinal walls in small amounts and poses a health hazard in the body. If too much is taken, it will leak out of the rectum, creating an embarrassment for you.

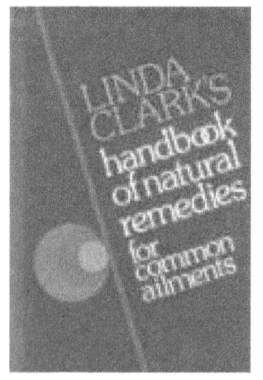 In her book, Linda Clark's Handbook of Natural Remedies for Common Ailments, Linda writes about mineral oil, "The message has finally got through to the public, and the medical profession that mineral oil is

one of the most damaging of all laxatives. It robs the body of Vitamins A, D, E, and K: It interferes with absorption of calcium and phosphorus, and can actually lead to other diseases."

Some of the lubricant drugstore laxatives are:

• Alin plus phenolphthalein

- Dioctyl sodium sulfosucciante – a detergent type substance that lowers the surface tension of your colon walls and fecal matter.
- Docusate potassium
- Magnesium hydroxide – brings in more water into your colon.
- Osmolak plus lactulose (lactulose is a synthetic sugar that pulls water out of your body and into your colon to soften stools.)
- Sokol plus mineral oil

Dioctyl sodium Sulfosucciante belongs to a family of chemicals that reduces the surface tension of the fecal matter in your colon. This allows water and fat to penetrate and make the fecal matter softer. These chemicals are known as,

- Dioctyl sodium succiante (also known as docusate sodium)

- Dioctyl potassium succinate (also known as docusate potassium)
- Dioctyl calcium succinate (also known as docusate calcium)

Health Alert: Again do not use mineral oil when using these types of succinate laxatives.

If you are pregnant, do not use mineral oil or other oils to get relief from constipation. During pregnancy, you need good absorption of minerals to provide nutrients for your newborn. Excessive use of mineral oil during pregnancy can cause bleeding in newborns.

Osmotic chemicals – Saline Carthertics

Osmotic chemicals are salts and other compounds that activate secretions of water from your colon walls and into your colon, which are absorbed by the fecal matter. This softens the fecal matter and promotes a bowel movement. These laxatives should be used only for a short time, since they can become habit-forming.

Health Alert: Osmotic laxatives promote bowel movements by bringing large amounts of water into your colon. In this bowel movement, minerals that body needs are also eliminated in the stool.

Here is a list of osmotic chemical laxatives you will find at the drugstore.

- Amphohgel
- Epson salt
- Maalox – contain aluminum and magnesium hydroxide
- Magnesium hydroxide

Milk of magnesia – is a saline laxative, which causes stools to hold fluid, which promotes peristaltic action. Magnesia can neutralize acids you need for digestion and can give you excess magnesium.

Sorbitol – is found in fruits and vegetables. It can also be created in your body through chemical synthesis. It can hold a large amount of water in your colon, making stools softer.

Health Alert: Do not use osmotic laxatives in high doses. They can be toxic and affect the kidneys. If you have weak kidneys do not use this type of laxative.

Stimulant Laxative Cathartics

Stimulant laxatives have strong laxative action and should be avoided, if possible. These laxatives stimulate your colon by irritating your colon walls. This irritation causes peristaltic movement. When these stimulants are used over a long time, they become habit-forming and can damage your colon wall by desensitizing cells and nerves along your colon.

These laxatives have some side effects such as nausea, cramping and diarrhea. But, not everyone will experience these side effects. Cascara Sagrada and Senna are popular herbs with strong stimulative action. Many other herbs also fall into this category.

It is always best to use these herbs when prepared by well-known companies. It is also best to use an herbal combination, since these herbs work together to provide colon toning, detoxification, cell building, and colon stimulation.

Health Tip: Use herbal combinations for five days or less. Just use them long enough to clear your constipation.

Some of the stimulant laxatives you will find at the drugstore are:

Cascara sagrada

Castor oil – not recommend since it will irritate your colon

Correctol – contains Bisacodyl

Dialose plus – contains phenolphthalein

Dulcolax – contains bisacodyl

Exlax – contains bisacodyl and sennosides

Feenamint – contains bisacodyl

Perdiem – contains senna

PeriColace – contains casanthranol

Health Alert: All laxative of any type can produce Diarrhea, if they are too strong or are used excessively.

If you use castor oil, make sure you take it little by little and not a lot, at one time. Castor oil is thick and can get stuck in your throat and cause you to gag.

Laxatives, if abused, produce electrolytic imbalances, sodium excess, esophageal blockage, diarrhea, and constipation.

Health Alert: Bisacodyl interferes with absorption of potassium in your colon.

Some Drugstore Laxatives contain various chemicals and compounds such as belladonna alkaloids – atropine, scopolamine. They contain Nux vomica a form of strychnine, a rat poison. They also contain podophyllum and aloin, which produce strong bowel action making them unsafe.

Health Tip: If you have been on a drugstore laxative, try one of the Natural Laxative Methods or Herbal Laxative Combinations in this book. Add to this more fiber food.

When using strong laxatives, your entire colon can be quickly cleaned out. This means your next bowel movement will not occur for 24 hours or longer. So don't panic thinking you are still constipated.

5: What You Should know about Your Colon

One feature of your colon is the lack of nerve sensors that give you pain, when your colon is not working correctly. It is only after a lengthy time, that any colon disease shows itself and only after it has progressed into a serious illness.

This is why constipation, though just a colon symptom, should be a warning, you need to pay attention to. Your colon is central to your entire health. Constipation is a major sign your health is at risk.

In David Webster's book, acidophilus and Colon Health, he points out that,

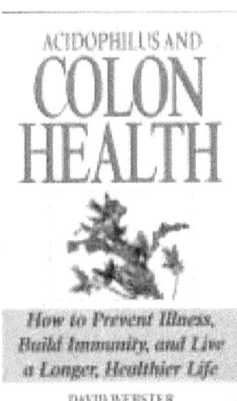

ACIDOPHILUS AND
COLON
HEALTH

How to Prevent Illness,
Build Immunity, and Live
a Longer, Healthier Life
DAVID WEBSTER

"Today, science knows your colon as much more than an organ of elimination. It plays an important role as part of our immune system and in absorption of nutrients into the body. It influences liver, brain, and nerve function, and directly affects the function of other organs of elimination such as the kidneys, urinary bladder, lungs, and skin. The health of our colon determines the health of our bloodstream, organs, tissues, thus also affecting our immunity and longevity."

The health of your colon revolves around the survival and domination of good bacteria. By keeping your colon saturated with good bacteria, you can expect good colon health and little trouble with constipation. But, you have to include some good lifestyle practices.

But before discussing good bacteria, let's look at your gastrointestinal tract, starting at your mouth.

Gastrointestinal Tract

When the food you eat reaches your colon, it has passed through many digestive processes. These processes start at the mouth with pre-digestion of carbohydrates and proteins. They end with re-absorption of minerals and water in your colon walls, from your fecal matter.

Formation of mucus

What happens when you eat meats and processed foods? Eating meats, eggs, dairy products, cream, ice-cream, cheese, milk, bread, flour products, and food in bags or packages cause a formation of mucus that appears in the throat, colon and throughout your body.

If you wake in the morning with mucus and congestion in your throat, you are eating too many processed foods.

Mucus Membrane

The lining of the gastrointestinal tract, which runs from the mouth to the rectum, is called mucus membrane, or mucosa. This lining protects the tissue below it from all types of contaminates, pathogens, or poisons that enter through the mouth and nose. It does this by excreting a mucus slime, which absorbs contaminates or irritants then moves them out through your rectum.

Mucus Slime

This mucus slime is produced when meats or processed foods you have eaten irritate the lining of the gastrointestinal tract. This mucus slime is produced in any part of the body that rejects food by-products it cannot use. This mixture of mucus and unusable byproducts are stored on tract walls, in organs, joints and tissue.

When the time is right, this mucus slime comes out of your body, when you have a cold, flu, diarrhea, constipation, and other illnesses that have discharges.

This mucus slime is damaging to the internal membranes, joints and organs. It coats and sticks to internal membranes and causes them to malfunction and weaken overtime.

In your colon, mucus slime coats the walls of your colon and eventually hardens as it collects other pasty and sticky residues from your fecal matter.

This mucus slime decays and becomes toxic overtime. This creates an environment favorable for bad bacteria, by creating an alkaline environment. This colon condition then readily produces constipation.

Mucus slime is created throughout your body in the internal tract lining. This lining occurs in the stomach, intestines, colon, throat, ears nose, eyes, liver, veins, arteries, bladder, kidneys, heart, vagina, lungs and respiratory system. This slime interferes with the way the stomach, intestines and your colon work, by blocking absorption of nutrients into the body.

In the small intestine

By the time food you have eaten reaches your colon, at least 90% of it has been digested and absorbed through the small intestine walls. The rest is cellular waste, undigested or undissolved foods mixed to become chyme.

Realize that not all that has been absorbed through the small intestine is good. If your intestinal walls have been damaged, by eating too much junk food, then bad nutrients, poisons, food particles, free radicals, and other junk can move into your blood and body, where it creates mucus slime.

Chyme

As your food enters your small intestine, it is called Chyme.

Chyme consists of liquid, fiber, minerals, and various other waste products. Chyme consists of,

- Bile

- Cellular and tissue waste

- Cholesterol

- Food wastes

- Mineral ions

- Living and dead bacteria

- Mucus

- Toxins

- Undigested fats

- Undigested fiber

- Water

Bile

Bile is also found in the fecal matter. What is bile? It is a liquid that is produced by the liver. The liver excretes bile into the gallbladder, where the gallbladder stores it.

When food reaches the duodenum, the start of the small intestine, a sensory agent triggers the release of bile from your gallbladder and digestive juices from the pancreas. Bile and digestive juices then travel to the duodenum. There they help to make your digested food acidic. In addition, these digestive juices help to break up fat globules into tiny droplets that can be easy digested.

Bile pH is alkaline and in the range of 7.1 to 8.5. The juices from the pancreas have a pH of 7.2 to 8.2. These alkaline secretions serve to neutralize acid in the small intestine (Any pH above 7.0 is alkaline and any pH below 7.0 is acidic.)

Bile consists of,

- Cellular and tissue waste

- Cholesterol

- Food wastes

- Mineral compounds of sodium, potassium, calcium

- Living and dead bacteria

- Mucus

- Toxins

- Undigested fats

- Undigested fiber

- Water

- Mucus

Liver, Gallbladder, Pancreas

The liver, gallbladder, and pancreas have a major role in small intestine digestion and colon adsorption. When these organs do not create the needed secretions, food is improperly digested and absorbed. When you don't digested correctly, you will not create the nutrients required for good colon function.

So, no matter how healthy you eat, if your small intestine or colon do not function right, you can still be malnourished.

Small Intestine – Cecum Connection

The end of the small intestine is connected to the start of your colon call the cecum or lower part of your colon. This connection has a valve, which controls how much chyme enters your colon or cecum. This valve is called the ileocecal, (il'e-o-se'kal) valve. This valve must work properly, otherwise it can lead to poor health conditions. If the valve closes slowly, it can allow more chyme into your colon before it is ready.

Under these conditions, the chyme might have too much water causing you to have diarrhea.

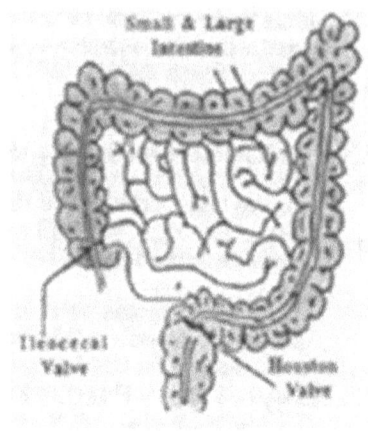

When the ileocecal value is weak and does not close tightly, colon bacteria and fecal matter can slip back into the small intestine causing a bacterial overgrowth. This overgrowth, in the small intestine, can cause severe diarrhea and poor absorption of fats soluble vitamins such as A, D, E, and K.

After chyme enters the cecum, the lower part of the ascending colon, the ileocecal value closes. This value should remain closed, but if it does not, fecal matter could be sucked back into the small intestines and migrate into the common hepatic duct and liver. This results in toxins being pulled into the blood, which contributes to various disease states.

Health tip: When the ileocecal valve does not close properly, the valve tone and tissue show weakness. To avoid this condition and to keep this valve strong, massage the area on the right side just above your pelvic bone and near your appendix.

RUB your ILEOCECAL VALVE DAILY to strengthen and tone its tissue.

Rub the ileocecal valve when you are in the shower. With your fingers and soap, rub the valve area for about 15 seconds or so daily.

Soap and water lubricate your skin, so your hand can flow easily on your skin. Push down slightly in the valve area and make a rotating motion, while your fingers remain stationary or move slightly.

Colon Function

Around 4-5 % of the food you eat gets absorbed in your colon.
Some of the roles of your colon are to absorb water, mineral ions, and vitamins from the fecal matter and to move this ionic liquid through the lumen, gut wall, into the blood vessels. When this takes place with little or no toxins being absorbed through your colon walls, the body's immunity improves.

When water is absorbed through your colon

walls, it is re-circulated back into the blood and into the lymph system. The re-absorbed mineral ions move into the lymph liquid and then into the cells to feed and build body organs and tissues.

If toxins are also absorbed into the bloodstream, they weaken the body by making it acidic and causing all sorts of unpleasant symptoms or diseases. Eating fruits and vegetables offset the acidic effect.

Your colon has many other functions to perform:

- Absorbs vitamins through your colon wall - created in your colon by friendly bacteria and move these vitamins into the bloodstream – riboflavin, nicotinic acid, biotin, folic acid and vitamin K.

- Absorbs inorganic solutes, chemicals, and moves them into the blood to be detoxified by the liver

- Eliminates the mucus cellular waste from the lymph system

- Forms bulk and compact fecal matter
- Houses millions of good bacteria
- Keeps pathogenic bacteria and pathogen at bay
- Keeps a pH of 6.2 – 6.8.
- Moves fecal matter through your colon
- Removes excess cholesterol and estrogen from the body
- Uses fiber to start peristalsis movements.

Large Intestine

Your colon, also called the large intestine, is part of the gastrointestinal system, which starts at the mouth and ends at the anus. Your colon consists of the following:

- ileocecal valve
- cecum, appendix
- ascending colon
- transverse colon
- descending colon

- huston valve

- sigmoid

- rectum

- anus

Cecum – Appendix

Once in your colon, chyme is called fecal matter. The fecal matter moves passed the ileocecal value and into the cecum. By peristalsis action, the cecum moves the fecal matter into the ascending colon.

If the fecal matter sits too long in the cecum, fecal matter can move into the appendix just below the cecum. When this fecal matter is not moved out of the appendix through peristaltic action, the appendix can become toxic and form bowel pockets. These pockets can become infected, leading to appendicitis.

As the fecal matter sits in the ascending colon, and as it is squeezed to move it further into the transverse colon, water is removed from the fecal matter.

The longer fecal matter sits in the ascending colon the more water is removed from this matter and the harder it becomes. The longer fecal matter sits in any part of your colon the more protein putrefies, carbohydrates ferment, and fats become rancid.

As food rots in your colon, more toxic gases are formed. These gases get into your bloodstream, your organs and joints. They cause discomfort and disease, if you are exposed to them over a longtime.

HERE IN THE ASCENDING COLON – fecal matter moves upward to the transverse colon. In constipation, it is in the curve of your colon where it changes from the ascending colon to the transverse colon where fecal matter frequently piles up.

When the transverse colon turns into the descending colon, fecal matter can pile up, at the turn. These are the areas where massages would be helpful, in helping the fecal matter to move forward.

In the ascending colon, water and ionic minerals are also removed from the fecal matter, and it starts to harden. As the fecal matter travels through your colon, its consistency will harden. If it does not have fiber and other ingredients that hold onto to water. Most processed foods have little fiber, and therefore, they lead to constipation.

IN THE TRANSVERSE COLON – more water minerals are absorbed from the fecal matter, and the fecal matter becomes firmer.

HERE IN THE DESCENDING COLON – less water and minerals are absorbed, and the fecal matter is being stored for later release from the rectum.

HERE IN THE SIGMOID COLON - fecal matter is held until it is ready to be released through the rectum by the Huston valve. When the fecal matter is held here too long, it starts to accumulate. This causes the sigmoid to expand, balloon, or
become distorted.

HERE IN THE RECTUM – fecal matter is stored until you have the urge for a bowel movement.

The Huston valve is at the end of the sigmoid colon and opens into the rectum. When the Huston valve is weak excess, fecal matter moves into the rectum. This may cause you to leak fecal matter into your clothing or have a bowel movement when you are not ready.

Health Tip: To keep the Huston valve strong and healthy, so it open and closes when it should, rub it from the outside at the same time you rub your ileocecal valve. The Huston valve is found on the left side of your body straight across from the ileocecal valve.

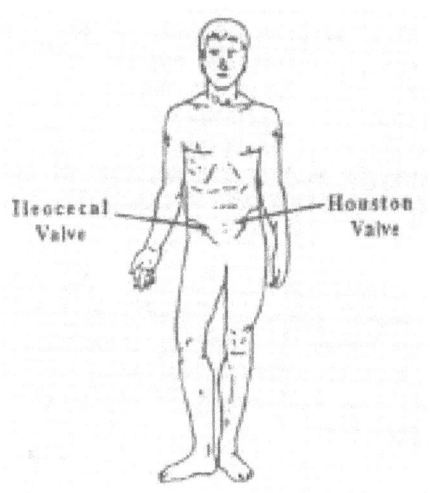

If the Huston valve does not open when it should, then fecal matter will stay in the sigmoid colon and create constipation.

Micro Flora in Your Colon Bacteria in your colon are referred to by many different names – probiotics, good or bad bacteria, beneficial bacteria, acidophilus, disbiosis, and micro flora, pro flora, friendly flora, and unfriendly bacteria.

The terms good and bad bacteria are used in this book to refer to all the bacteria that exist in the small intestine and your colon.

Your colon has both good and bad bacteria. The good bacteria maintain the health of your colon by keeping the bad bacteria from multiplying.

Most people have bad bacteria as the dominant condition in their colon. You can see this by the illnesses that exist throughout the world. Most people later in their lives suffer from diseases that resulted from colon neglect and abuse.

Bad bacteria multiples, when you consume poisons, such as pollution, pesticides, food additives, and,

- Drink alcohol

- Eat processed foods

- Have excess anxiety

- Lack fiber in your diet

- Use birth control pills

- Use drugstore laxative

- Use drugs and medication

Good bacteria in your colon consist of hundreds of species of bacteria. The good bacteria are most active in a pH of 5.9 to 6.9- an acidic environment. This makes for a healthy colon.

Your colon serves as a home for good bacteria, which ferments specific carbohydrates. This fermentation keeps your colon environment slightly acidic. The acid environment favors good bacteria and keeps the bad bacteria and pathogens from multiplying.

The bad bacteria create an alkaline environment and are most active in a pH of 7.1 to 7.9.

The good bacteria create an acidic environment and are most active in a pH of 5.9 to 6.9.

Acidophilus and Bifidus are the main good bacteria that exist in your colon. The ascending colon has the most bacteria. The quantity of bacteria becomes less in the transverse colon and lesser in the descending colon. Eventually, little bacterium is found in the sigmoid and rectum.

When good beneficial bacteria are dominant, in your colon, it prevents the spread of disease from various organisms –parasites, bacteria, viruses, and fungi. The specific organisms are,

Shigella, salmonella, viruses, encephalitis, protozoan, amebas, staph, herpes, flu and cold viruses, comphylobacter, and CMV, which create killer diseases such as dysentery, blood poisoning, meningitis, pneumonia, influenza and encephalitis.

The good bacteria keep these organisms in the minority, thus preventing them from multiplying, getting into the blood and into different body organs. They do this by their antibiotic like secretions, lactic acid production, and other secretions, which keep their environment acidic.

The good bacteria live and thrive on carbohydrates. When your body has good digestion and little carbohydrates reach your colon, the good bacteria population decreases, and the bad bacteria become dominant.

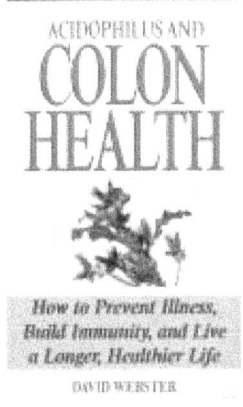

Good bacteria need to be fed to keep them dominant in your colon. If there are any good bacteria left in your colon, then by feeding them, you can get them to multiply. If there are not any good bacteria in your colon, then you cannot reestablish the good bacteria, by eating specific carbohydrate foods. To reestablish good bacteria, under this condition, you must do a flora enema.

In his book, Acidophilus and Colon Health, 1999, David Webster, also says, "Indicators of a healthy colon flora are a soft but well-formed stool, with amber color and little or no odor, and that floats in water most of the time. When the stools are dry, dark brown, too solidly formed or too loose, and especially if there is a putrid odor, these are clear indicators of a putrefactive, alkaline-producing colon flora.

Chronic constipation, diarrhea, and irritable bowel syndrome are often eliminated when your colon is restored and maintained at a slightly acidic pH."

In his research, Webster found that feeding the remaining good bacteria edible lactose whey rejuvenates the good bacteria in your colon. By drinking 2 – 5 tablespoons or more each day in a cup of distilled water, enough lactose can reach your colon to feed your good bacteria. Webster recommends doing this for 30 days. After this period, you can check your stools to see, if you have reactivated your good bacteria.

To get more information on Edible-grade whey search for David Webster on Google.

If you are allergic to lactose or milk products, then you can use FOS, fructooligosaccharides and syrup. FOS is useful for constipation, since it acts like a fiber and stimulates peristaltic movement. FOS is not digestible, so it will reach your colon where the good bacteria use it as food. It also has the ability to increase absorption of minerals in your colon.

FOS are long chain fruit sugars, is found in fruits and vegetables. Those highest in FOS are onions, leeks, oats, garlic, Jerusalem artichoke, barley and rye.

Look for FOS Products on the Internet, in case you're allergic to milk products.

In Robert Gray's research, he has found three foods that help feed the good bacteria and help to keep your colon pH acidic. He prefers using vegetables because they are nonmucus forming foods.

1. Onions – eat at least one medium-sized onion each day. The onion can be eaten cooked or raw.

2. Cabbage – eat cabbage or drink cabbage juice. Drink at least 3/ 4 cup of cabbage juice three times a day and eat at least one pound of fresh organic cabbage each day. This amount is necessary to provide the good bacteria with plenty of food to get it to multiply. Cabbage has an added advantage of suppressing the bad bacteria.

3. Sun Choke or Jerusalem artichokes – eat 4 oz. of sun chokes each day. Sun chokes contain a carbohydrate call inulin, which is not digested or absorbed in the small intestine. This allows it to reach your colon where it feeds the good bacteria.

Bad Bacteria Domination

When you have constipation, your bad bacteria will multiple and in a time, move into your small intestine. When this happens, food in the small intestines is digested less and become fermented causing gas.

The bad bacteria are pathogen, disease producing, and thrive in an alkaline condition. This bad bacterium lives on undigested protein and causes it to putrefy. It produces ammonia, as it uses up protein, which neutralizes some of the surrounding acid, making the environment more alkaline.

This bad bacterium tends to become dominant in your colon, since carbohydrates are digested better than protein, making more undigested protein available for the bad bacteria.

Good and bad bacteria cling to the walls of your colon. Sometimes they move into the wall cell structure and live inside.

Good Bacteria Domination

Good bacteria are dominant in your colon when it is 85% of all the bacteria in your colon. When the bad bacteria are more than 15% of all bacteria in your colon, then the bad Bacterium is becoming dominant, and your colon starts becoming toxic and disease prone.

Good bacteria in your small intestine and colon have many functions:

- Helps digest milk and nutrients
- Suppresses the bad bacteria by keeping pH levels in your colon acidic.
- Reduces cholesterol levels
- Produces B vitamins
- Keeps your colon walls strong, so they can perform
- peristaltic movement
- Helps to prevent constipation

- Eliminates toxic chemicals

- Helps to eliminate gas

- Keeps the immune system up

Acidophilus and all other good bacteria in capsule or liquid form must be stored in the refrigerator. But, there are capsules that are designed for storage at room temperature.

Other Parasites

Your colon is also a place for other organisms to breed and live. Many are harmful to your health and enter the body in various ways – foods we eat, through the bottom of your feet, air you breathe, the water you drink, and through sexual activity.

What do we find in your colon? We find single cell protozoan, molds, parasites, fungus, viruses, bacteria, worms (round worms), and yeast (candida albicans.) By eliminating constipation, eating more fruits and vegetables, cleaning and detoxifying your colon, you can rid yourself of many parasites. There are herbal formulas that will help you purge these unwanted organisms out.

Now, don't think you don't have parasites and other organisms in your colon. It is reported that 1 in 6 people have parasites in their body.

Symptoms created when you have parasites are not always clear-cut. Occasionally, there are no symptoms. So, doctors are not always able to say when your symptoms or illnesses are created by parasites. You can suffer from parasites for years, without knowing why you don't have good health or feel run down all the time.

Some common types of parasites are:

- **Round worms** – can be up to 14 inches. You can get round worms by eating improperly cooked meat or by handling dogs or cats infested with round worms.

- **Tapeworms** – can be acquired by eating improperly cooked beef, pork, and fish.

- **Pinworms** – are mostly found in children who get them from other children by touching their infected clothing, toys and dirty hands.

- **Giardiasis** – is a protozoan that is common among travelers. This parasite is found in untreated water, contaminated food, and can be transmitted sexually.

- **Bistoplasma capsulatum** – is an infectious fungus that is found in dirt or in soil. This fungus can cause lung diseases.

Health tip: There are many good parasite remedies such as olive leaf extract, black walnut, wormwood, and grape seed extract. If you have bloating, loose bowels, excess gas or other gastrointestinal conditions, try taking olive leaf extract or a drop or two of grape seed extract each day.

Gastrointestinal Transit Time

Transit time is the time it takes food to move from your mouth to your rectum. A reasonable time is 16-22 hours. Three ways to check your transient time is to:

Eat corn and leave some corn un-chewed. Check your stools to see when this corn comes out. First thing in the morning, drink one oz. of chlorophyll with 8 oz. of distilled water and the juice of one lemon. Eat breakfast and then check how long it takes to see green stools.

Drink some beet juice with your next meal. See how long it takes to see red stools.

6: Fruit Juice Remedies That Reduce Constipation

Fruit Juice Constipation Remedies

Look at the different remedies listed in the different following chapters and use the one that feels right for you. Maybe it is the one where you have all the ingredients. Or, it could be the one you are familiar with the ingredients. You may combine a few and see how that works for you.

Ok let's get started. We are going to start listing the ways you can get relief from your constipation. For those who have been constipated for three to five days, you can use any of the methods listed. And, since your constipation is considered severe, you will have to use a combination of the remedies listed.

Keep in mind that even the simplest method can work even with chronic or severe constipation. Each one of you is different and will react differently with specific remedies.

For Difficult Constipation Cases

For more difficult cases of constipation, sometimes more than one remedy might be necessary to relieve your constipation. From the list that follows you can use one remedy and if this does not work keep using this remedy but start using a second.

For Mild Constipation Cases

For cases of mild constipation, it may take a day or so to get your bowels moving again. For a more moderate case, it may take 2-4 days. For a severe case, it may take a week or so, since your bowel wall may be weak and needs toning.

Health Alert: If you use natural foods with laxative effects, their
laxative effect diminishes after long-term use.

Health Alert: If you have diabetes or adrenal fatigue, limit your use of fruits and juices, when you first wake up in the morning. However, exercising in the morning will help you tolerate drinking some juices in the morning.

Organic Juices

Organic fresh made juices have cleansing and laxative action. These juices contain loads of mineral, bioflavonoids, vitamins, enzymes, antioxidants, and other nutrients. Citric fruits have citric acid. And, the more tart they are the more acid they have.

Fresh juice is a fast way to get all types of nutrients into the blood quickly. As juice nutrients get into your blood, they suck out toxics and build up tissue. In your colon, they destroy bacteria, feed wall tissue, pull out toxins, and activate peristaltic action.

Health Tip: Even though juices provide helpful action throughout the body, it is best to limit their use and drink them in larger quantities, only when trying to accomplish certain health benefits.

When juicing fruits and vegetables, the more fiber that is left in the juice the better results you will get with your constipation.

It is always best to use fresh juices, but as a last resort, using packaged juices will be better than not drinking anything. Try to buy juices that are in a glass container and not plastic.

Method 1: Apples and Apple Juice

Apples are good for eliminating constipation, because they are high in pectin, a soluble fiber. They have many minerals, and contain Sorbitol - a natural sugar, which stimulates peristaltic action. Pectin helps to detoxify the intestines and promote regular bowel movements.

The fiber in apples adds weight and bulk to your fecal matter and helps draw water from your colon into the fecal matter. This keeps your stools from becoming hard and difficult to eliminate.

Apples are one of best fruits to eat, because they are high in minerals, which provide alkaline electrolytes to your body. What this does is neutralize acids that are created during illness, anxiety, anger, exercising, breathing pollution, and improper eating. Body acid is the major reason we get deadly diseases, as we age.

Make eating apples or drinking fresh apple juice a daily habit. Eat them as snacks between meals. They are also effective in liver and gallbladder problems.
Here's what to do.

Use crisp and hard apples such as granny smith, fuji, or gala for juicing.

Drink three glasses of apple juice each day, morning, noon, and evening. In combination with drinking fresh apple juice, eat 3-4 apples each day to get fiber.

One-day apple and apple juice fast

You can also do a one-day apple and apple juice fast by, Eat 3-4 apples during the day. Drink apples juice every hour.

Don't eat anything until the next morning. Then, start changing your eating habits as listed in later chapters.

If you do not want to do a one-day fast, then eat your apples and drink fresh apple juice morning, noon, and night.

Apple cider vinegar

Take 1-2 tablespoons of apple cider vinegar with 8 oz. of water every day. And, add apple cider vinegar to your salad as part of your salad dressing. Just adding it to your salad will help to kill any bacteria or parasites that are in your vegetables. Apple cider vinegar will also kill any bacteria or parasite in your stomach that can cause you to have diarrhea.

Apple and Pear Juice

Prepare equal amounts of fresh apple and pear juice. Drink this combination, when you first wake up and one hour before bedtime.

Juice the pears that are slightly hard. If the pear is ripe, blend it whole with apple juice to create a thick drink. Using the whole pear will give you additional fiber. Just remove the seeds, but do not peel it if it is organic.

Pears have minerals, vitamins, and chemicals that help to clean out your colon, and kidneys. Use them to regenerate your blood cells.

Method 2: Apple Juice and Prune Juice

If you have a juicer, you can make fresh apple juice and drink 3-4 glasses a day. You can also drink store-bought apple juice, but try to get fresh squeezed and not the type that has been flash pasteurized or pasteurized. If you can find fresh apple juice, then use flash pasteurized.

Buy your juice in glass containers. Plastic containers are processed using solvents that stay in the container walls and gradually outgas into the apple juice. This out gassing is more severe when plastic containers are stored in hot places.

To speed up the laxative effects of apple juice, take the following combination first thing in the morning before you have breakfast,

- Drink 2-3 cups of prune juice

- After ½ hour, drink one cup of apple juice

- Then, 1-hour later drink another cup of apple juice

Be prepared to head for the bathroom, after you drink your prune juice and your first glass of apple juice. You may need to head to the bathroom soon after you drink prune juice, everyone is different. Keep drinking apple juice every hour until you have a bowel movement.

Prune juice by itself is good for constipation. It is a safe, gentle and an effective laxative. Drink a cup in the morning and a cup in the evening. Prune juice contain the substance **dihydrophenylisatin,** which is responsible for the laxative action. Prunes are also high in iron and are a great supplement, if you are anemic or low on iron.

If you add prune juice to your diet, do not drink as much of it as you would when you have constipation. Drink ½ glass in the morning and perhaps ½ glass in the evening. After a month do not use it any more, for a while. Excess use of prune juice will make its laxative effects less effective.

Method 3: Apple Juice, Figs and Raisins

Here's another recipe using apple juice. Use it the first thing in the morning before breakfast.

In a blender, put in a cup of fresh apple juice. Add equal amounts of dry or fresh figs and raisins. Choose how many figs and raisins to use. You will need to experiment a little. Get a consistency that is not too thick. Add a little more apple juice, if needed.

Method 4: Oat Milk with Fig Juice or Prune Juice

Buy oat milk at the health-food store. In the morning, warn 8 oz. of oat milk and add the following:

- 3 oz. of fig juice or prune juice and two droppers full of licorice extract.

- Or you can mix one glass of 50% fig juice and 50% prune juice.

Drink this first thing in the morning.

Method 5: Stewed Figs

Take 10 – 12 calimyrna figs and stew them in two glasses of water (16 oz.) for 10 minutes. Let them sit in this water overnight.

In the morning remove the figs, warm and drink the juice. Eat the figs though out the day.

Or prepare a blended drink of,

- three or more figs, fresh or sun dried

- one banana

- 1 tablespoon of honey or molasses

- one cup of rice dream

Drink first thing in the morning and any time after lunch or dinner.

Method 6: Mulberry Juice

Mulberry juice has many health benefits. It is good for digestive tract illnesses. It can stimulate digestion and assimilation of nutrients in the small intestine. It is useful for older people for reliving constipation.

Mulberry contains many minerals and vitamins.

Method 7: Berries and Cherries

Boysenberry

Boysenberry juice has a gentle natural laxative action on your bowel. When your constipation is mild, this juice will help move things in your colon.

Blackberries

Mix ½ cup of distilled water and ½ cup of blackberries. Drink this first thing in the morning to promote peristaltic movement.
Drink this often and it will make you regular.

Blackberries are high in vitamin C.

Cherries

Cherries are high in antioxidants, fiber, potassium, and many other minerals, which are effective in neutralizing body acid. Cherries contain vitamins B-1, B-2, folic acid and niacin.

Cherries have laxative effects and can start peristaltic action.
Eat fresh cherries throughout the day or drink three 8 oz. glasses of cherry juice during the day.

Buy cherry juice in a glass container.

Elderberry Juice

Elderberries can be used to help reduce the symptoms of colds, flu, and diabetes. It also helps to relieve constipation, diarrhea, and hemorrhoids. Drink 1–2 glasses each day. Increase the quantity if necessary.

Method 8: Citrus Juices

Citrus juices are an excellent way to stimulate your colon and other parts of your body. Since your colon is less active at night, drinking juices as soon as you awaken and get up can stimulate strong peristaltic action and promote a bowel movement.

Lemons

Lemons are filled with minerals, especially potassium, Vitamin C, and bioflavonoids. They have a cleansing action for the entire body. They help you get rid of mucus inside the body and have a cleansing effect on your blood.

Fresh lemon juice is the king of fruit juices. It contains citric acid, which acts on your body in a way no other juice does. First, it acts on the liver to build up its enzymes, so it can detoxify toxins in your blood. Then, it combines with calcium to form soluble chemical substances. This makes it effective in removing kidney and pancreatic stones, plaque buildup along artery walls, and other calcium deposits that occur in your body.

When your liver, gallbladder, and pancreas are not working right, food digestion is affected. This in turn will create constipation.
Use lemons moderately, since they break up oils during digestion. In your body the make oils less available for your cells and joints.

Health Alert: If you have lemon allergies or ulcers, then you should avoid lemon juice. If you have arthritis, lemons are not a good choice.

Here's what to do:

Squeeze one lemon into a glass of warm distilled water. Drink it first thing when you wake up. Don't drink anything else for at least 1/2 hour.

You can use a citrus press to juice the lemon or just squeeze it, to get the juice out.

Grapefruit Juice

Instead of drinking lemon juice, drink a glass of fresh squeezed grapefruit, first thing in the morning. Again wait at least 1/2 hour before you eat anything.

Health Drug Alert: If you are taking any anticonvulsant drugs, birth control pills, estrogen, protease inhibitors and even other types of drugs, avoid drinking grapefruit juice. It slows the breakdown of certain drugs, allowing them to increase in the blood to dangerous levels.

Grape fruit and Orange Juice

In the morning combine grapefruit and orange juice. Just prepare a half-and-half drink of these citrus fruits and drink it, first thing in the morning. Place it in a thermos and drink it throughout the day.

Method 9: Pineapple Juice

Drink a glass of pineapple juice, first thing in the morning. Don't eat anything for at least half an hour. Then drink another glass at noon and just before you go to bed. Do this for the next three days. Experiment by adding other citrus juices to the pineapple.

Method 10: Coconut and Carrot Juice

Mixing fresh coconut and carrot juice provides a tasty drink that has good laxative effects. Experiment with the amount of juice you want to mix, according to your taste. Drink this mixture for three days.

7: Fruit Remedies That Activate Your Colon

Fruits the Perfect Food

Fruits are made by nature and are a perfect food. They contain the right balance of nutrients with distilled water. You gain enormous benefits from eating fruits, especially if you eat the outer skin. They should be eaten without cooking. They are easy to digest and absorb and do not stress your colon.

Fruits contain fiber, which help to cleanse your colon and prevent constipation. Most fruits help provide the body with minerals that help your body reduce acid, as it is created. And most important of all, fruits help cleanse the body of mucus slime that accumulates throughout the body.

Fruits do not leave any slime residue in your body when eaten, except when they have pesticides and preservatives in their outer skin. They do not ferment or putrefy in your colon, as do processed foods, dairy products and meats.

Choose your fruits carefully. They should be eaten when they are fully ripe. Do not eat them, if they are under ripe or overripe. In the under ripe condition, they may be acidic and in the overripe condition, the many contain excess natural sugar.

Fruits, vegetables, and grains contain fructooligosaccharides, FOS. It is this compound that helps to feed the good bacteria in your colon. Without an adequate supply of FOS, good bacteria will dwindle and bad bacteria will flourish.

Method 11: Just Plain Fruits

Eat fruits throughout the day, during breaks, and especially in the evening. This will help you promote a bowel movement, in the morning.

These are the fruits you should eat.

- Apples

- Apricots

- Avocados

- Bananas
- Blueberries
- Boysenberries
- Cantaloupes
- Cherries
- Figs and dates
- Grapes
- Lemons
- Papayas
- Peaches
- Pears
- Persimmons
- Plums
- Prunes
- Raspberries

Apples

Eat 3-4 apples a day to relieve constipation. Both gala and Fuji apples are good, since they are small and crisp.

It is best to use fresh organic apples. When eating apples as a snack, since you will not know what pesticides were used in growing the apples. If apples are not organic, it is better to peel the apple, before eating.

Using baked apples also helps to clear constipation.

Eat one baked apple at night, right before bedtime, and in the morning. Do this until your constipation is cleared.

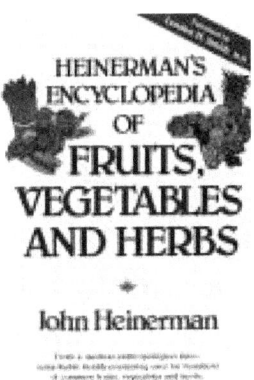

In his book, John Heinerman, Heinerman's Encyclopedia of Fruits, Vegetables and Herbs, describes how to bake apples: "Cut apples in half and clear out the centers. Add chopped dates to the center. Pour some cranberry juice over the dates and apples. Then sprinkle cinnamon and nutmeg on the top. You can pour cranberry juice on some of the apples and see if you like the taste after they are cooked. Cook apples for 46-60 minimum, at 375- 400 C."

Dried Apples

Dried apple slices are also a good source of fiber. However, when the slices are dehydrated most nutrients are lost, but fiber is retained. Sulfur dioxide is typically used to dry apple slices, and this can cause allergic or asthmatic reactions in some people. It is not recommended to use dried apple slices in place of fresh organic apples.

Just Apples and Mineral Water

Just after waking, eat two unpeeled apples, chew well, and then drink 8 oz. of water that has two drops of Alkalife, or a squeeze of lemon juice. Or, you can use any other mineral additive or supplement you use.

This combination of apples and activated mineral water will stimulate your colon to become less sluggish and to move fecal matter out of the rectum.

You can find Alkalife on e-Bay. This product cost $29.00 on the Internet, but it can be bought it for $17.00 on e-Bay.

Apricots

Apricots are one of most nutritious fruits, since

they are high in fiber, vitamin A, C, potassium, and minerals. One apricot has around 1000 IU of vitamin A. This vitamin is mainly in the form of the precursor beta-carotene.

Apricots have a laxative effect and are usually available during the summer. Dried apricots are also good and are much higher in vitamin A and in minerals.

Use dried apricots that have not been dried with sulfur dioxide. Some people are allergic to sulfur dioxide and it is considered a pollutant that is found in our air. This chemical is a preservative that prevents apricots from turning brown.

Health Alert: If you have an ulcer, eating apricots with sulfur dioxide can increase your stomach acid and aggravate it.

Avocado with Apple Cider Vinegar and Lemon

Here's a recipe that will make you go to the bathroom in a couple of hours.

- Peel 1-2 avocados
- Add a little sea salt

- 3-4 tablespoons of apple cider vinegar (to taste)

- 1-2 tablespoons of lemon (to taste)

Mix all together and spread on your favorite crackers.

Have a good time eating

Yes, avocados are high in fat, but it contains the fat that is good for you, monounsaturated. Half of an avocado contains 500mg of potassium and folate.

Bananas

Bananas are rich in potassium. They assist in healing open wounds in the interior body membranes. They are helpful in stopping diarrhea and at the same time in promoting bowel movements.

Eat two bananas on an empty stomach followed by a glass of distilled water. After your constipation is cleared, eat only one banana each day.

Blueberries

Blueberries can act as a laxative for some people despite its use to stop diarrhea. These berries have chemicals, anthocyanosides that can kill bacteria and viruses.

Blueberries are also excellent for reducing inflammation. This makes them good for inflammations that occur all along the gastrointestinal tract.

Boysenberries

Boysenberry juice has a gentle natural laxative action on your bowel. When your constipation is not extra serious, this juice will help move things in your colon.

Cantaloupe

Cantaloupe is one of the best fruits you can eat. It contains many minerals and has Vitamin A and C. It is high in potassium. It has plenty of fiber and is useful for constipation. Mix them with watermelon, to get the extra water.

Cherries

Cherries are high in potassium, fiber, and many other minerals, which are effective in neutralizing body acids. They contain vitamins B-1, B-2, folic acid, and niacin.

Cherries have excellent laxative effects and can start peristaltic action. Eat fresh or dried cherries throughout the day or drink 3 glasses of cherry juice, during the day.

Figs and Dates

Figs are high in fiber and can provide a gentle action on your colon, when you are constipated. This action can take about 24 hours, before it takes place.

The use of figs and dates combined can have a stronger action on your colon.

You can find fig syrup **on the internet to use in some of the smoothies you make.**

Grapes

Grapes have a good laxative action. Eat 1-2 lbs. of grapes though out the day, and reduce the amount of food you eat, during the day. Eat more vegetables and other fruits. Reduce the amount of processed foods you eat.

Grapes are high in vitamins and minerals. They have good fiber content and are especially high in manganese.

Since they are high in sugar, bugs are attracted to them and farmers to spray them with pesticides. Try to find them at the farmer's market as organic or not sprayed.

Papaya

Papaya is well known for its enzyme papain that helps you digest protein. Its minerals help reduce cell waste and eliminate stomach and colon mucus. Use this fruit in your smoothies.

Persimmon

Eat 2-3 persimmons each day, if they are available. They will help keep you regular.

Plums

Fresh plums are filled with minerals and have a mild laxative effect. They can relieve gas and have a cleansing effect on your intestines.

Prunes

Prunes are dried plums. Eat both for their natural laxative effect. Prunes are more effective than plums for constipation. Buy a bag of dried prunes and eat them throughout the day. Aside from this laxative effect, prunes are high in iron.

You can also soak prunes in water over night. In the morning put the water and prunes into a blender with a little apple juice and blend them. Drink this as your morning drink.

8: Vegetable and Juice Laxatives

The benefits of Vegetables

Juices, with their nutrients, are absorbed quickly into your bloodstream. As a result, your cells are provided quickly with nutrients that feed them and wash away waste. Juices give you the opportunity to get quick relief from various body conditions, such as constipation. Juices move into your colon quickly to cleanse it and to activate peristaltic action.

The Benefit of Minerals

Eating and drinking vegetable juices provide you with minerals and nutrients that build your blood, tissue, bones, and cells. It is minerals that build every part of your body. It is minerals that keep your body's pH at the required level. It is minerals that keep your body alkaline by neutralizing body acids.

It is minerals that build your colon wall tissues and cells, so your colon can perform those activities that prevent constipation.

Vegetable Juices for Constipation

So, let's look at which vegetables and vegetable juices can help you end constipation.

Keep in mind that some natural recipes for clearing constipation require drinking vegetable juices that are bitter or have a strong taste. As you will find, some of the vegetable juices taste good and some don't. Remember, you are dealing with a condition that needs clearing and that what you drink for this is not for always for pleasure.

As you drink some of these vegetable juices, you may find that you like certain ones and these can become your regular daily or weekly drink.

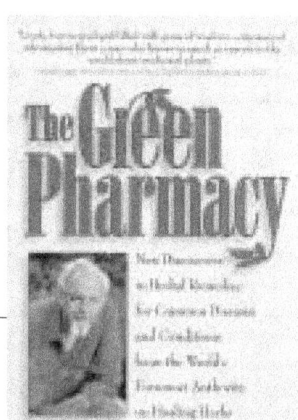

James A. Duke, PhD, in his book, The Green Pharmacy, gives the following constipation remedy using rhubarb.

"Rhubarb has strong laxative action so it is best to use it with other juices. Here's how you can use this herb. Blend together three stalks of rhubarb, without leaves, 1 cup of fresh apple juice, and one quart of peeled lemons and one tablespoon of honey or maple syrup. This tart drink will help you with your constipation. Drink one glass three times a day."

A smaller quantity of this rhubarb drink would be,

Blend three stalks of rhubarb, ¼ - ½ peeled lemon, a teaspoon of maple syrup, and ¾ cup of fresh organic apple juice. You may add more syrup, if the taste is too harsh for you. Don't use rhubarb leaves since they contain toxic chemicals.

Health Alert: Use rhubarb only raw, since it is high in oxalic acid. Use it sparingly and do not cook it. Cooking converts the organic oxalic acid into inorganic oxalic acid. The body does not easily absorb inorganic oxalic, and it forms crystal deposits in the kidney and throughout the body.

If you have arthritis or gout, do not use rhubarb.

Method 12: Carrot Juice

Carrot juices contain certain oils that work on the mucus membranes of your stomach and colon. This helps with digestion and starts your bowels functioning properly. Carrots are high in fiber and beta-carotene, an antioxidant, which the body converts to vitamin A. Carrots can make your stools softer and larger.

Why are larger stools better? Because larger stools dilute toxins, exposure fewer toxins to colon walls, and press against colon walls to promote peristaltic action.

Drink carrot juice twice daily, once in the morning and in the evening, before bedtime. You can drink more carrot juice, if you like. Its action on the body produces enormous benefits, since it contains a good number of vitamins and minerals – B, C, D, E, K, carotene, sodium, and potassium. These nutrients help to clean out your colon and speed up fecal matter movement.

As you increase the carrot juice you drink, chances are you will feel a little uncomfortable. This happens when carrot juice reaches your intestines and colon and begins stirring up the toxic layers and matter in that area. This feeling will pass and is nothing to worry about.

Health Tip: If you are pregnant, drink carrot juice daily to build up your breast milk and to provide your baby with the nutrients that it needs.

Method 13: Carrot Juice, Carrots and Celery

An effective way to clear constipation is to combine vegetables that are high in fiber and that have laxative effects.

Celery is high in fiber, potassium, sodium, and many other minerals. It can reduce inflammation and protect against cancer. Celery has a chemical call polyacetylene, which reduces prostaglandins that cause inflammation.

Celery has a calming effect on the nervous system. If you have been using laxatives, which have overworked your colon nerves, celery will help to relax these nerves and give them a rest.

Adding carrot juice to celery juice provides an even better nutritional drink. This drink will help to restore nerve function, in your colon. Celery has the highest content of organic sodium. This sodium is used throughout the body as lymph saline liquid allowing cells to work and live properly.

Celery is also beneficial for the stomach. The stomach lining is filled with sodium and this sodium necessary to prevent ulcers. The stomach is considered a sodium organ.

Here's what to do,

Eat carrots and celery, during the day and in your salads; drink a glass of carrot juice in the morning and one in afternoon. By eating slightly steamed carrots you can increase the carotene available from the carrots by up to 4 times. However, by cooking carrots, you destroy the enzymes that will help you to digest them quickly and completely.

Boost your carrot juice by juicing with it a few stalks of celery, which includes the leaves. The leaves have more nutrients than the stalk and are part of the nutritional value of celery.

Tomato, Carrot, Celery Drink

Here's a drink you can take in the afternoon to activate a bowel movement.

With a juicer, juice some tomatoes, carrots, and celery. By experimenting, you can discover the amount of vegetables to use, according to your taste.

Mostly likely you will want equal amounts of tomatoes and carrots, and you will want to add a few stalks of celery, including the leaves.

Now, let's add a few more items to give your drink more pushing power. Squeeze in a small amount of garlic, onion, and radish. While juicing your carrots, juice a small bunch of spinach or parsley.

Drink 1 to 1 ½ cups in the morning.

Method 14: Carrots, Cabbage and Raisins

Because carrots contain fiber, they help to form a good stool and promote peristaltic action. By combining carrots with cabbage and raisins, you can create an even more powerful food that will help in relieving constipation.

Combine the following vegetables to form an evening salad:

- Chopped carrots
- Shredded cabbage (raw or slightly steamed)
- Romaine lettuce
- Cauliflower
- Cucumbers
- handful of raisins
- Sprinkle a tablespoon of grounded flax seeds
- Mix in 1 – 2 tablespoons of olive oil
- Mix in 2 tablespoons of apple cider vinegar
- One tablespoon of lecithin granules

Eat this salad once or twice a day for three days. After that you should continue eating a vegetable salad for lunch or dinner.

Method 15: Carrot and Spinach Juice

Combine 10 oz. of carrot and 6 oz. of spinach juice. Drink two pints daily. Both these vegetables have nutrients to help relieve your constipation.

Cucumber

Cucumbers are good for preventing constipation. However, they can be used in the carrot-spinach juice or the apple-spinach juice.

Cucumbers make these juices more powerful. Use only about ¼ - ½ of a cucumber when adding it to these juices. You can experiment with how much cucumber you want to add.

Cucumbers are a natural diuretic and help to dissolve kidney stones. Because they are high in potassium, they help to promote the flexibility of colon cells. This helps to keep your colon working, as it should.

Method 16: Cabbage and Asparagus

Cabbage is high in fiber and contains a good amount of potassium, beta-carotene and many other nutrients – bioflavonoids, indoles, genistein, and monoterpenes. It is these different chemicals that give it its potent ability to reduce or prevent colon cancer and heal various ulcers along the gastrointestinal tract.

Cabbage is anti-bacterial and helps to heal tissues in the stomach, intestines, and colon. Drinking cabbage juice produces intestinal gas. This gas occurs, when cabbage juices combine with putrefied layers in the intestines and colon.

Health Tip: Use little or no salt on any preparation of cabbage. Salt destroys the nutritional value of cabbage.

There are many forms of cabbage you can use for your juices – green, red, savoy, and bok choy

Asparagus

Asparagus are high in fiber and provide vitamins A and C. Refrigerate asparagus quickly, if you are not going to use them and keep them for 3 days or less. Asparagus that have not been refrigerated lose their nutritional value quickly.

Health Alert: People with gout should not eat asparagus, since they contain purines that can start a gout attack.

With a slight amount of water, steam for 3-4 minutes, cabbage and asparagus in a glass pot. Eat just before going to bed.

Beets

Beets are high in fiber, organic sodium, potassium, Vitamins A and C, iron and calcium. If you like beets, eat 2 raw beets in the morning and expect to have a bowel movement 10-12 hours later.

Method 17: Cabbage and Beets

Blend 1/3 part beets and 2/3 part cabbage. Drink this mixture on an empty stomach. This is a strong tasting drink, but the cabbage contains a cleansing enzyme, lysozyme, which absorbs bacteria and toxins. This toxic material is eventually moved out in your fecal matter. Beets also promote bowel movements.

Cabbage and other juices

To make cabbage juice tastier, mix it with celery stalk and leaf juice, tomato juice, and a citrus juice or pineapple juice. This juice can be used in the morning or evening. Or, make a cabbage soup with ginger.

Method 18: Sauerkraut Juice

Sauerkraut juice is a natural remedy and used by many people, who have been constipated.

In their book, Home Remedies What Works, Gale Maleskey and Brain Kaufman, discuss sauerkraut juice.

"I've used sauerkraut juice many times to relieve constipation of five or six days' duration, and it has always worked for me,' says Jacqueline, 49, a Floral Park, New York, housewife. She picked up the remedy from her father, who used to drink sauerkraut juice regularly. 'He lived to be 86 years old and never had any health problems,' she says.

She simply drains the juice - usually about ¾ cup – from a large can of sauerkraut, and then drinks it. 'For me, it works as well as milk of magnesia. I can count on results in about 1 to 1 ½ hours.' She's not alone. Several other people said sauerkraut juice is an effective laxative"

Health Alert: Sauerkraut juice should not be used regularly, since it is high in salt. The salt helps to pull water into your colon, which helps to relieve constipation. In this process, electrolyte minerals are also flushed out. Regular use of sauerkraut can deprive the body of vitally needed minerals and cause a health problem.

Sauerkraut and Tomato Juice

Perhaps a more tolerable drink, using sauerkraut, is to prepare it as follows:

Mix equal parts of sauerkraut and tomato juice. Add a touch of lemon and drink this twice a day, once in the morning and then in the evening.

Method 19: Sweet potatoes

Sweet potatoes can help you become regular. Prepare sweet potatoes, just before you go to bed. Boil or bake the sweet potatoes. Then eat them with some add milk, some salt, and honey. This mixture for sure will get your bowels moving the following day.

Corn

Cook corn for about 5-7 minutes. Don't overcook it. This will provide you with a great source of fiber. Eat more cooked vegetables, until your constipation is cleared. But, be sure to cook them for a few minutes to soften them slightly. Cooking them too long makes the fiber soft and less effective in your colon.

Method 20: Greens

In her book, Healthy Digestion the Natural Way, Berkson outlines a base for a "tasty green" recipe.

It has been have changed it slightly, to make it more powerful for relieving constipation.

In a pan add some water with one or more teaspoons of olive oil. Turn the heat on and sauté some garlic. Now add small pieces of chopped broccoli. Cover and cook for around two minutes. Next add a bunch of spinach, chard, collard greens or kale, which ever green you like. Cook for a few minutes. Add some water or oil as needed.

Serve with a pinch of apple cider vinegar, lemon juice, or balsamic vinegar. Add a bit more olive oil, or flax seed oil.

This provides an excellent source of fiber, chlorophyll, good oil, and minerals, to help clear your constipation.

Health tip: When using flax seed oil do not heat it. Use it only at the end of the heating cycle, when you are ready to eat your food.

Another Green Remedy

In boiling distilled water, add mustard greens, collard, chard, and turnip leaves. Any three will do. Allow this mixture to cool slightly. Then eat the greens and drink the water. This will promote a bowel movement.

Endive Leaves

Endive lettuce has a bitter taste. However, its juice is good for clearing constipation. Use this juice in small quantities, with other juice mixtures. Mix it with a carrots, spinach and apples.

Method 21: Radish with Sesame oil

For constipation, mix 2 tablespoons of grated radish with 1 tablespoon of sesame oil or with one-tablespoon of tamari soy sauce. Take this once or twice each day, to clear your constipation.

Parsnips

Parsnips contain more fiber than most other vegetables. This makes them ideal for helping clear your constipation. Use the small parsnips, since they are softer than large ones.

Parsnips are also high in potassium and contain chemicals that neutralize carcinogens, in the small intestine and colon.

9: Fruits - Vegetables That Create Peristaltic Action

Method 22: Apple Juice and Spinach Juice

Here's a recipe that is found in Heinerman's Encyclopedia of Healing juices, 1994. Heinerman says to, mix equal parts of apple juice with spinach juice.

Use one or two small apples and one bunch of spinach. Spinach may or may not have a strong taste for you, so use apples accordingly. Use two apples or more, to make this drink tasty.

Take two cups each day, one in the morning and one in the evening. Continue taking this mixture for about two weeks. After this time, evaluate how you feel and decide if you want to continue taking this mixture. If so, use this drink at a reduced interval – twice a week or once a week.

What you may experience with this mixture is after 3-4 days of use, your bowel movements in the morning may come out in 3 seconds, and that's it; you're ready for your shower.

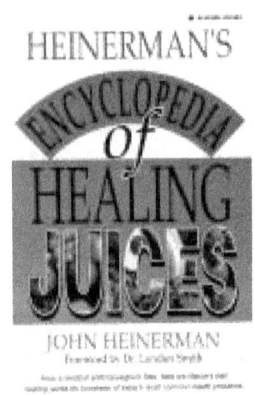

Here's what Heinerman says about this apple and spinach combination, "I've put many clients on two cups of this apple- spinach juice each day for up to a week and have had testimony after testimony come back to declare how the most difficult cases of constipation, which no laxatives could begin to touch, had suddenly cleared up within a matter of days!"

In addition, Heinerman claims that this juice combination has a cleansing action on your bowel walls. It helps to remove some of the encrusted fecal matter that has collected on your colon wall, over the years.

When it is cooked, raw spinach juice is high in oxalic acid, which binds with calcium in the body. Even though you use it uncooked, in this recipe, I still recommend you take a calcium supplement, with this apple and spinach combination.

It is recommended that you use 1:1 magnesium: calcium combination of about

1000 - 1200 mg. For good intestinal absorption of these minerals, use Calcium Aspartate, Calcium Lysinate, Calcium Citrate or a combination of all three. Most combinations you find in health-food stores provide these minerals in a 1:2 combination. But, if you look hard enough, you will find a 1:1 magnesium:calcium supplement.

N.W Walker D.Sc., in his book, Fresh Vegetable and Fruit Juices, 1978, says,

"Organic oxalic acid is one of the important elements needed to maintain the tone of and to stimulate peristalsis...oxalic acid in our raw vegetables and their juices are organic, and as such are not only beneficial but essential for the physiological functions of the body. The oxalic acid in cooked and processed foods, however, is definitely dead, or inorganic, and as such is both pernicious and destructive.

When the Oxalic acid has become inorganic by cooking, then this acid forms an interlocking compound with the calcium even combining with the calcium in other foods eaten during the same meal, destroying the nourishing value of both. This results in such a serious deficiency of calcium that it has been known to cause decomposition of the bones. This is the reason that I never eat cooked or canned spinach."

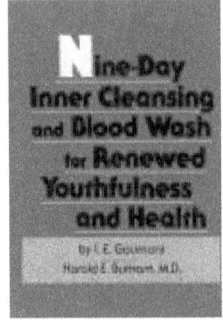 I.E. Gaumont and Harold E. Buttram, M.D also recommend spinach for constipation. In their book, Nine-Day Inner Cleansing and Blood Wash for Renewed Youthfulness and Health, they say, "SPINACH is a protective food, particularly for the glands. A high source of vitamin A, and rich in chlorophyll, it is helpful in high blood pressure, functional heart trouble, anemia... It is indicated in medical circles that raw spinach juice taken in quantities amounting to about one pint daily has often corrected the most aggravated case of constipation in a short period of time."

Spinach is the riches plant source in folic acid and shortage in this vitamin can create constipation. It is also high in antioxidants, such as beta and alpha carotene, lutein and zeaxanthin. It also contains potassium, magnesium, vitamin K.

Celery, Spinach, grapefruit drink

Here's another juice drink you can make, using spinach. Mix a combination of spinach, celery, and grapefruit juice. Drink this first thing in the morning.

Method 23: Sauerkraut and Grapefruit Juice

This is a fast working remedy, if you have a blocked colon.

Drink 8 oz. of warm sauerkraut juice

Follow this with 8 oz. of warm grapefruit juice

Be ready to head for the bathroom. If this fails to rush you to the bathroom, try this combination again, 45 minutes later.

You can also use just plain sauerkraut for constipation. Eat sauerkraut each day for 5 days each week.

10: Herbal Constipation Remedies You Should Know

Herbal Remedies

Chickweed

Drink 1 cup of chickweed every 3 hours. Do these until you have bowel movement.

Method 24: Chinese Rhubarb

Chinese rhubarb, rhubarb, turkey rhubarb has been used for many decades, to relieve constipation in China. It has a strong purgative action – it encourages strong laxative stimulation. It should be combined with other herbs, which reduces its purgative strength.

Health Alert: pregnant women should not use Rhubarb.

Rhubarb, Ginger, licorice Infusion

For severe constipation, prepare an infusion of,

- 1 teaspoon of rhubarb powder

- ¼ teaspoon of ginger root

- ¼ teaspoon of licorice root

Drink 1/2 cup of this infusion and over a few days increase it to a cup.

Bentonite

Bentonite is clay from volcanic ash. It is used to cleanse your colon walls and can be used as a laxative. You will see it as an ingredient, in some natural laxative formulas.

Method 25: Butternut Root Bark

Butternut root bark is considered one of the safest laxatives. This following formula is a gentle, but effective laxative herbal combination.

- Butternut root bark

- Cascara Sagrada bark

- Rhubarb root

- Ginger root

- Licorice root

- Irish moss

- Cayenne

This combination, with butternut, is listed in a book called, The Scientific Validation of Herbal Medicine, 1986, by Daniel B. Mowrey, Ph.D where Mowrey say,

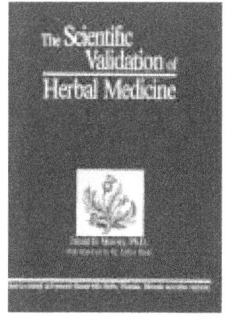

"This combination is due to the effectiveness of Butternut Root Bark – a mild and effective laxative – and Cascara Sagrada – one of the most effective herbal laxatives around and in addition helps to return the natural tone of your colon. Ginger Root contains an oil called Ginerol which helps to bind the other herbs together and deliver them into your colon which they can assist in normalizing your colon."

Chamomile Tea

Chamomile tea is often used as a relaxant and is useful in reducing tension, which can lead to a tight colon. It has a gentle laxative action and helps in digestion.

Drink one cup just before bedtime.

Method 26: Cayenne

Cayenne is effective in producing colon peristalsis, by aiding in digestion and stimulating elimination. It can be used regularly or when needed for constipation. Cayenne pepper is known to help thin the blood. So, it is good for improving the blood circulation.

Cayenne is available in capsules of different strengths, from 5,000 heat units (HU) to 100,000 and even higher.

In addition, cayenne when used with other herbs helps to deliver these herbs more efficiently to where they are needed in the body.

Health Tip: Start with one capsule of 40,000 HU and always take it after you eat. You will feel a hot or slight burning feeling in the upper stomach and that's when you know it is working. This burning sensation will pass, as your body gets used to digesting it.

Health Alert: Do not use cayenne seeds, as they can be toxic. If you are pregnant or breast-feeding do not take cayenne supplements. Use cayenne only as showed on containers and only as capsules.

Health Drug Alert: Cayenne has the ability to block the ulcer producing effect of NSAIDS. It also has shown to increase the body's absorption of theopylline, a drug used to treat asthma.

In his book, Left for Dead, Dick Quinn tells how Cayenne pepper saved his life after coronary bypass surgery failed to restore it. In this book, Shannon Quinn, say,

"One of the most effective stimulants, mostly, cayenne targets the digestive and the circulatory system. Cayenne regulates blood pressure, strengthens the pulse, feeds the heart, lowers cholesterol, and thins the blood. It cleanses the circulatory system, heals ulcers, stops hemorrhaging, speeds healing of wounds, rebuilds damaged tissue, eases congestion, aids digestion, regulates elimination, relieves arthritis and rheumatism, prevents the spread of infection and numbs pain."

Use the recommended dose shown on the bottle, of cayenne you use.

You can also add cayenne pepper into other foods. Add cayenne to soups, salads, and other food you like.

In soups or salads, break open a cayenne capsule and mix it in. You can add 1 – 2 capsules but first start with 1/4 or 1/2 capsule, so you can get use to the hot taste. Start with ¼ capsules, when adding it to soups.

If you are pregnant, it is considered safe to use cayenne.

Web Link for The cayenne pepper formulation created by Dick Quinn.

http://www.cayennecompany.com/catal og/heartfoods/

Method 27: Cascara Sagrada

Cascara Sagrada comes from the bark of the buckthorn tree. It stimulates your colon to produce stronger contraction than normal. It can work on the most difficult cases of constipation.

It is one of the best herbs with a strong laxative effect. It will be found in many herbal combinations that are mixed for constipation.

Cascara has Chrysophanic acid, which stimulates your colon wall to produce peristaltic action. Cascara also contains a chemical called emodin, which controls the strong action of Chrysophonic acid, thus producing a balanced laxative effect.

If you use cascara in an herbal mixture, do not use this mixture for more than thirty days. Then take a rest from it. Do not use cascara in large amounts and for long periods since it can cause intestinal distress and become habit-forming.

Cascara Sagrada also stimulates secretions from the liver, gallbladder, pancreas, and stomach. These secrctions give cascara additional laxative effects.

Health Alert: Do not use Cascara Sagrada if you have irritable bowel syndrome, hemorrhoids, or ulcers. Use Cascara for a limited time. It can become habit-forming and if used for an extended time, it can increase the risk of colon cancer. Its use also causes you to lose potassium with each bowel movement.

If you have liver problems do not use cascara sagrada full strength. Use it in combination with other herbs. Cascara is known to put a strain on the liver.

You can take cascara as a single herb. As a single herb, it can cause cramping and nausea. However, used it with other herbs. In an herbal combination, the combination can detoxify your colon, and colon walls, cleanse the blood and produce other synergistic actions.

Senna Tea

You can also prepare a senna tea as follows:

Buy some senna tea at a health food. Place a tea bag into 1 ½ cups of distilled water and steep. Then, add the peel of a whole red potato. Also, add a couple slices of potato meat. Add to this, a teaspoon of wheat or oat bran and flax seed.

Simmer this combination, strain it and drink the liquid. This will help some of the more difficult cases of constipation. Remember the longer you simmer this combination the stronger the tea will be. Start with a 5-10 minutes and then work up to 15-20 minutes. But, you need to experiment with the time.

When you drink senna tea, drink only 2-3 oz. at a time and drink it only after it has cooled down. It has less of a cramping action when you drink it cool.

Senna Tea with Mint

Here is another senna tea you can prepare.

- 1 teaspoon of senna tea leaves
- ½ teaspoon of peppermint leaves.

- Boil 8 oz. of distilled water, turn the heat off, and stir in the herbs. Turn the heat off and cover the glass container. Let tea simmer for 3-10 minutes.

- Add honey to improve taste and some powered vitamin C if you have it.

Health Tip: Look for formulas that have a small amount, 1/10 of a part, of fennel, anise, or ginger to reduce any cramping that might occur with senna.

Health Alert: Do not drink senna tea or capsule if you have any type of colon disease, stomach pain, diarrhea, or are pregnant.
Senna Pods are milder than the leaves since the do not contain resin. It is the resin in the senna leaves that causes griping in your colon.

If available, use around 8 pods. Heat some distilled water. Place the pods into the water for 5-10 minutes. Strain the tea and add 3-4 dried prunes or chopped prunes. Let cool and eat the prunes during the day or drink and eat a few prunes just before you go to bed. Drink only a couple ounces of the senna liquid, at one time. If cramping or griping occurs, reduce the amount of tea you drink.

Method 28: Psyllium

Health alert: If you have asthma, do not take or use psyllium. Some people with asthma have had allergic reactions to psyllium seeds and their powder.

Some you may be allergic to psyllium. If you are, you may become constipated or develop dark areas under your eyes.

Psyllium is the fiber part of seed husks from plantain. It is high in a soluble fiber that is called mucilage, so it absorbs water and becomes bulky. It contains almost no insoluble fiber, yet it acts like it has both soluble and insoluble fiber. Stomach enzymes do not easily breakdown psyllium, so it moves into your colon, like insoluble fiber.

In your colon, psyllium activates peristaltic action and helps to clean your colon of any stagnation that has occurred there. By adding moisture to dry hard fecal matter, psyllium helps to move fecal matter through your colon. As psyllium seeds bulk up in your colon, they push against your colon walls stimulating peristaltic action. The soluble fiber in psyllium provides food for good bacteria, which help them to multiple.

One added benefit of psyllium is its ability to pull toxins out of bowel pockets known as diverticula's.

Psyllium is a popular ingredient found in many natural and drugstore remedies.

Choose a psyllium product that does not have sugar, maltodextrin, or artificial sweeteners. If possible, buy psyllium in bulk form, from a health-food store, which may offer it in bins. In this form, it is processed less and usually contains no additives.

Here's how to use it:

For mild constipation, take one **tea**spoon in a glass of juice or warm water 3 times a day.

Health Tip: Work up to taking one teaspoon of psyllium by starting with ¼ teaspoon in a glass of water or juice, the next-day ½ teaspoon and so on until you are taking one teaspoon. Do the same when considering taking up to two teaspoons of psyllium.
Start by taking one **tea**spoon just before going to bed. After drinking your glass of psyllium seeds, follow this up, each time, with another 8 oz. of clear distilled water.

For moderate constipation, take two **tea**spoons in a glass of juice or warm water daily. Start by taking two **tea**spoons at breakfast time.

It can take up to three days to get relief, and that depends on the dose you take.

Use psyllium seeds with care. Some cases have been found where psyllium seed parts have lodged in your colon wall, causing an irritation. When using excessive psyllium seeds, it is possible that they can deposit on your colon wall, if your colon walls are coated with toxins.. This adds to the encrustation along your colon wall.

Health alert: When using psyllium seeds, drink water during the day, up to eight glasses a day. This helps push the seeds through your colon, so they don't deposit along your colon walls. Remember the seeds bulk up and absorb water and you don't want them to cause constipation, by bulking up and getting stuck in your colon.

Health Tip: Use psyllium seeds only long enough to relieve your constipation. Excessive use of psyllium can cause allergic reactions and can cause constipation, if used incorrectly.

Agar-Agar and Psyllium seeds

Agar and Psyllium seeds are mostly soluble fiber, which absorb a lot of water and bring it into your colon. This creates bulk in your colon, which puts pressure on your colon walls and creates peristaltic movement.

In his book, The Encyclopedia of Natural Health, 1962, Max Warmbrand, N.D., D.O.,

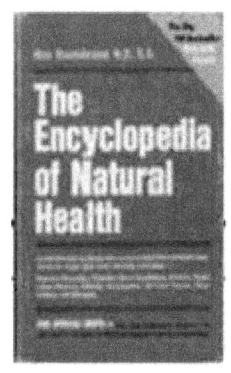 recommends that, "Remedies containing agar-agar or those manufactured from psyllium seeds or other water- retaining substances are often used to relieve constipation.

These remedies act up your colon because of their build, and because they absorb a great deal of water, which is then carried into the large intestine. We do not object too strenuously when these remedies are used to meet a temporary need, but must stress the fact that while they provide relief, they will not correct the underlying weaknesses which can be done only through the use of good foods, corrective exercises, and a rational way of living."

Agar-agar is seaweed, which is also known by other names —dai choy goh or kanten. Like psyllium, it is mostly soluble fiber. One disadvantage of these fibers is that once they form their bulk in your colon, they hold in nutrients that should be absorbed through your colon walls.

Agar is useful in improving digestion, pulling

toxins out of your colon and reducing hemorrhoids.

Method 29: Ginger

Ginger acts like a transporter to deliver herbs to a specific organ. It contains oil called **Ginerol**. It is a resin type oil that binds to other herbs in an herbal formula and helps delivers them to your colon. If a particular herb works on a specific organ, then ginger acts like a transporter to deliver that herb to that specific organ.

Ginger can stimulate your colon to peristaltic action. It can be used as capsule or as tea, to keep your bowels moving. In difficult constipation issues, ginger can be used as an enema and at the same time taken as a capsule. It is a gentle colon stimulant.

Ginger is best used in combination with other herbs such as cascara sagrada or rhubarb root. Ginger reduces the discomfort of these strong laxatives and helps to strengthen weak colon walls.

Health Tip: Ginger has not been tested to determine its effects on pregnant women. It may not cause a problem, but it is best not to take ginger while pregnant. You should consult with your obstetrician before taking it.

In the book, 10 essential herbs, 1992, Lalitha Thomas gives the ginger combination to relieve constipation.

"Chop one oz. fresh Ginger root or one tablespoon of Ginger power if the root is not available. Add to this 2 Tablespoons of whole flax seeds. Simmer in 2 cups of distilled water for 15 minutes. Add honey, unsulfured molasses, or pure maple syrup to taste."

Thomas recommends drinking 1-2 cups of this tea daily and points out that it is safe for children to use but half of this dose.

Method 30: Kyolic

Kyolic is a special garlic preparation, which is aged for 20 months in stainless steel tanks. With this aging, garlic odor is eliminated and certain chemicals are enhanced – S-allyl-mercaptocysteine, S-allyl-cysteine. These chemicals are powerful sources, for fighting cancer, heart and liver disease.

Kyolic cleanses, soothes, and reduces inflammation throughout your gastrointestinal tract. It is rich in potassium, which is necessary colon wall contraction.

Kyolic is also effective in killing pathogens and bad bacteria that live in your colon and elsewhere in the body. It also binds to heavy metals and other toxins that exist in the blood and colon and sweeps them out of the rectum. Aside from helping in constipation, it is helpful for reducing,

- fungus and other bacteria in your ear
- skin lesions due to bites or insect stings – use liquid form
- arthritis – requires 12 capsules a day
- diabetes – requires 12 capsules a day.

You can buy it in capsule and liquid form. Capsules are easy to take and have no side effects.

Here's how to use it,

For mild cases of constipation, take 2 tablets once or twice a day. For moderate cases, take 2 tablets three times a day
For severe cases, take 2 tablets five times a day.

Or if you prefer you can take 4-5 Kyolic capsules just before going to bed.

Continue this until your constipation is cleared. You can combine this Kyolic remedy with the apples and spinach remedy to help rebuild and remove toxic material, which is built up along your colon walls.

Continuous use of Kyolic is not harmful. It is the allicin in garlic that provides the stimulation to your colon to produce peristaltic movement.

Kyolic can be bought in health-food stores or on the Internet. You can type in Kyolic into the Google search engine to find where you can buy it.

Health Drug Alert: Garlic has blood-thinning abilities. Using it with blood-thinning drugs, pentoxifylline, NSAIDs is potentially dangerous, since excessive blood thinning can increase blood- clotting time. Do not use 3 days before any surgical procedure.
Garlic can also cause an allergic reaction or an upset stomach in some people.

Do not use garlic, if breast-feeding. Garlic can get into the breast milk, giving the baby colic.

Method 31: Aloe Vera

Health Alert: Menstruating or pregnant women should not use Aloe Vera, in any form, as a laxative.

Aloe Vera is a wonder herb that has been around for thousands of years. It has been used for both external and internal problems – skin rashes, burns, ulcers, and internal bleeding. It also promotes bowel movements, which help to relieve constipation. Some people are allergic to Aloe Vera. So, if you show a rash or have any undesirable symptoms, do not use it.

Aloe is an astringent, acts to tighten muscles, and has purgative and laxative action – dispels fecal matter that has collected in your colon. There are many aloe vera gel products to choose from. For best results, choose an aloe gel that is close to that of fresh organic aloe vera, whole leaf gel.

Take two tablespoons of pure aloe vera gel mixed with apple juice. You can use other types of juices that fit your taste.

If you use aloe juice drink, mix 1/3 of aloe juice with 2/3 of a juice you like, just before bedtime and just on awakening.

Marshmallow Root

Marshmallow root is a gentle laxative and will move fecal matter out of your colon. Use marshmallow root as a tea.

- Boil one cup of distilled water.

- Stir in one heaping teaspoon of marshmallow root.

- Cover pot and let tea sit for 10-15 minutes.

- Then, strain the tea and drink it.

- Take one cup in the morning and one in the evening.

Method 32: Peppermint Oil

Peppermint is used to soothe the nerves and is useful in relieving constipation when it is due to cramping and anxiety. It contains oils that stimulate the release of bile from the gallbladder. It also improves the function of the cells along your colon walls.

Health Tip: Use peppermint oil as an enteric-coated capsule, so the capsule does not dissolve in the stomach, but in the small intestine.

In the small intestine and colon, peppermint relaxes the muscles and promotes the release of gas.

Recommended dose of peppermint oil is 1 capsule three times each day between meals. Use peppermint oil only as recommend on package.

You can also add 2 drops of peppermint oil in an 8 oz. of water and drink after a meal.

Health Alert: Peppermint oil contains menthol, which is poisonous, when an overdose is taken. Always follow the recommend manufacturer's dose. If pregnant, do not use the enteric-coated peppermint oil. Do not give peppermint tea or oil to young children.

Method 33: Golden Seal

Golden seal has the compound, Hydrastine that gives it antiviral and antibiotic properties. It is use to fight off different types of infections internally and externally.

You will see golden seal in some of the herbal formulas for constipation, because of its properties to soften fecal matter and to regulate liver functions. It stimulates digestion and bile production, which in turn promotes peristalsis. It also heals the mucosa, your colon wall lining.

Golden seal is considered one of the top 10 herbs in the herbal world.

Health Alert: Do not use Golden seal for more than a week. Do not use it, if you are pregnant. Check with your doctor before using it, if you have diabetes, glaucoma, cardiovascular disease, or high blood pressure.

Do not use more golden seal than the recommended dose. In large doses, golden seal may create cardiac arrest or respiratory problems.

Method 34: Chlorophyll

Chlorophyll is the green substance that occurs in all plant and is one of the most helpful substances you can add to your diet. It is the blood of the plants. It helps to strengthen and thicken your colon cell walls. It inhibits the growth of pathogenic bacteria, which can cause various diseases, and feeds the good bacteria.

It detoxifies the cells in your body and colon, which houses an unbelievable amount of toxic matter.

Chlorophyll will help to get your bowels moving by improving your colon function. Use chlorophyll with any of the other methods you use to clear your constipation.

Take 2 capsules of chlorophyll just before meals

For the liquid chlorophyll, combine 1-2 oz. chlorophyll, juice of one lemon, and 8 oz. of distilled water first thing in the morning. This combination should sit well in your stomach and should not give you an upset stomach.
You can also add one or two tablespoons of chlorophyll to a glass of one half orange and one half grapefruit juice. With this mixture, you will not taste the chlorophyll much.

Health Tip: Chlorophyll is considered safe for pregnant and lactating women.

Method 35: Triphala

Drink this tea just before bedtime.

- Barberry   2 parts
- Boldo or Dandelion 2 parts
- Cascara Sagrada   1 part
- Licorice   1 part
- Rhubarb Root 1 part
- Ginger or Fennel   1 part

Health Alert: Some times, herbs can interact negatively with medications to produce a side effect that can be dangerous. Check with your doctor, if you decide to take herbs while on medication.

Some herbs are not properly prepared in standard strength or quality and will not provide you with any benefits of the real herb. As you buy herb products, you will become familiar with the companies that produce quality organic products.

Children's Remedy- Cumin Oil

Place a drop of Cumin oil on your finger and let your child smell the oil. Do this just before bedtime. This should promote a bowel movement in the morning.

Using Certain Herbs

Health Tip: Certain herbs such aloe vera, buckthorn, cascara sagrada, frangula, and senna have powerful laxative action. The chemicals called anthraquinones activate this action. Use these herbs as a last resort, when trying to clear your constipation.

When these herbs are used too long they can become habit-forming.

Use these herbs, only if they have been aged. Fresh herbs of this type can irritate your digestive tract and cause vomiting and bloody stools or diarrhea.

11: Constipation Remedies Unknown to most Doctors

Minerals

Minerals help the body produce energy and build bones, blood and cells. They are found in the blood, lymph liquid, and cell walls. They help in nerve transmission and muscle contractions, in your colon. Minerals are used with vitamins and other nutrients to form compounds that are essential, for your body's health.

Your body cannot create minerals, so you have to get them from the food you eat or through supplements.

Vitamins

Vitamins do not provide energy for your body. They are not found in your tissue and they do not build cells. But they do help to convert the food we eat over to nutrients that our body can use. This means they help enzymes break down our food - protein, fat, and carbohydrates. They are used in many chemical reactions that occur in your body. Your body can make only a few vitamins.

Mineral and Vitamin Supplements

The various minerals and vitamins recommended here should be taken individually or as a multi-mineral complex or as a vitamin complex. Avoid a supplement that contains both vitamins and minerals. There is some loss in the effectiveness of individual vitamins and minerals, when they are combined in multiform. Use capsules for best results, since capsules are filled with powder. Capsules dissolve quickly and so does the powder.

Some hard, tablet supplements may not dissolve completely in your stomach or intestines and flow into your colon and out your rectum.

Minerals in Fruits and Vegetables

Minerals in produce are the best minerals for your body. These minerals are in the form that nature created and are exactly what the body needs. They are electo-magnetically charged and have a life force that is provided by the plant. This life force quickly decreases after the fruit or vegetable has been picked. Therefore, it is always recommended to eat fruits or vegetables soon after they have been picked.

Electrolyte Minerals

It is best to take liquid electrolyte minerals. In this form, minerals have an electrical charge and are ready for use by your body. Electrolyte minerals, when placed in your mouth, are absorbed quickly though your mouth's lining. They are also absorbed easily in the lining of your gastrointestinal tract, as they travel towards your colon.

Minerals help to electrify your body. They improve brain function, nerve activity, blood structure, body structure, and body calmness.

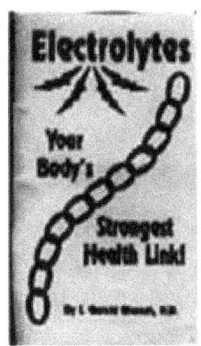 **Health Tip:** Add minerals to your diet by eating raw fruits and vegetables and through supplements. Minerals insure your colon has the proper tone and functions and this minimizing constipation.

In I. Gerald Olarsh, N.D.'s pamphlet called,

Electrolytes, he points out that, "Electrolytes in the body are minerals such as sodium, potassium, chloride etc. that are dissolved in the blood. When the electrolytes are dissolved they break apart into charged particles called ions.

The ions carry either a negative or positive charge. These charged particles create electricity that helps run the bodies of animals and humans. Electrolytes are the basis of good health because they are used in the maintenance and repair of all tissue, the utilization of amino acids, and as the basis of every physical and neurological function..."

The Next Best Mineral Supplements

If electrolytic minerals are not available, use chelated minerals. These minerals are attached to amino acids, making them magnetic, which allow them to flow right through the intestinal walls, without having to be digested.

Look for minerals such as,

Calcium aspartate

Calcium gluconate

Calcium Citrate

Magnesium glycinate

Selenium glycinate

Potassium gluconate

Mineral Absorption

Most minerals are absorbed in the last part of the small intestine and the beginning of the large intestine or colon. When your colon walls collect layer upon layer of waste, it affects absorption of the minerals you consume. When this happens, your body will be deficient in minerals and your appetite will be bigger than normal.

Method 35: Brewer's Yeast

Brewer's yeast contains all B vitamins, except B12. It also contains many other vitamins, minerals and is high in amino acids.
Brewer's yeast can help ease, reduce, or clear your constipation. If you can handle the taste, add it to your juices morning and night.

When you first use brewer's yeast, it will create gas in your colon. Brewer's yeast feeds your good colon bacteria, increasing their count. This increase activates a battle between the good and bad bacteria creating gas as a by-product. Keep using brewer's yeast until the gas stops. This many take a few weeks, but you are doing one of the best things you can do for your health – increasing good bacteria and reducing bad bacteria.

You can improve the benefit of using brewer's yeast, by eating cultured yogurt or taking good bacteria liquid or capsules, between meals. Do this between meals, so when you take your supplement your stomach does not put out too much HCl acid, which would kill the supplement.

Health Drug Alert: If you have gout or are taking monoamine oxidase inhibitors do not take brewer's yeast.

Method 36: MSM

MSM stands for methyl sulfonyl methane. MSM is organic sulfur. It provides many benefits for your body and is widely used as an anti- inflammatory and is especially beneficial for arthritis pain. MSM is used for all body cells and tissue, including joint tissue.

MSM in your colon stops or blocks the activity of cholinesterase (ko-li-nes-ter-ace.)
What is cholinesterase?

Our nervous system is composed of a network of nerve cells, which start at the brain and end on all parts of our body. It is nerves that direct muscle contraction or expansion. After the muscle completes its movement, an enzyme cholinesterase is released, which stops the muscle from moving again. Without the nerve signal blocking cholinesterase, the muscle would continue to move nonstop.

MSM is useful in clearing up constipation. When used at 6000-8000 mg each day, At these doses, you can expect 2-4 bowel movements each day. As MSM blocks the activity of cholinesterase, it allows more peristaltic action to occur in your colon. This results in more bowel movements.

By using 2000-4000 mg of MSM, you many experience 1 to 2 bowel movements each day. Of course, for each person the amount will be different.

The action that MSM has in your colon is useful for older people who have less nerve signal for peristalsis. Cholinesterase stops the few peristalsis signals older people have, thus creating constipation.

In S.W. Jacob, M.D., R.M. Lawrence M.D., Ph.D., and M. Zucker's book, The Miracle of MSM, 1999, they say,

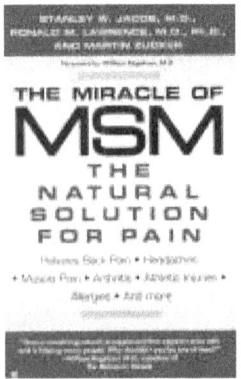

"As a dietary supplement, MSM offers great potential for anyone with constipation. MSM produces a general "tonic" effect upon the bowels and normalizes bowel function, particularly for older individuals.

We have given MSM to nursing homes, where constipation is a common problem. The nurses have said that MSM works well for patients, even for individuals not responding to Metamucil or stool softeners."

Rich distributing has good-quality products. Buy the 1000 mg MSM torpedo tablets. This allows you to easily take 4000-5000 mg of MSM, by only using 4-5 tablets. They are easy to swallow.

Health Alert: MSM has not been evaluated for effects during pregnancy, so it is best not to use it during this time.

Method 37: Vitamins

The following vitamins help in normalizing and clearing constipation:

Vitamin A

Vitamin A should never be taken by itself. It should be used with other vitamins or taken with food or with fruit snacks.

When taken alone, Vitamin A will putrefy in your colon creating toxic chemicals that may get into your blood.

Vitamin A helps to protect your mucous membrane along the gastrointestinal tract from bacterial attacks. It is also effective in reducing kidney and gallbladder stones.

Vitamin A is essential for a healthy liver. For some individuals, taking vitamin A daily would eliminate constipation.

Vitamin A is an important vitamin, which helps to improve your immunity. Since your colon is an important part of your immune system, it is recommended you eat those foods, which are high in Vitamin A or to use a Vitamin A supplement. Vitamin A will strengthen your colon.

Vitamin A also helps you absorb protein in your small intestine. Any protein that is not absorbed will move into your colon undigested. This undigested protein in your colon decays, producing highly toxic material that can cause serious illness over time.

Health Alert: If you are pregnant or planning to get pregnant, do not take more than 5000 IU each day of vitamin A, to avoid birth defects.

If you have any liver disease, consult your doctor before taking vitamin A.

Foods high in vitamin A are, Green leafy vegetables, carrots, eggs, yellow vegetables, butter, liver, cabbage, prunes, celery, parsley, spinach, kale, cheese, tomatoes.

The Mineral Magnesium

Jesse Lynn Hanley, M.D., in his book call, Tired of Being Tired, 2002, gives another way to take Magnesium to relieve your constipation, "Take at bedtime. Begin with 200

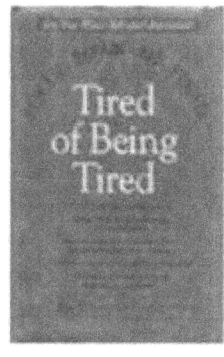

milligrams magnesium oxide or magnesium citrate—you may increase the dosage in200-milligram increments until your bowels move regularly. The dose for magnesium is individual, so begin low and increase the dosage as needed. Reduce the dosage if you experience loose bowels. Unlike irritating laxatives, magnesium does not create laxative dependency."

Health Drug Alert: If taking hypoglycemic drugs, magnesium may increase absorption of these drugs. It is recommended you consult with your doctor on the effects of magnesium, with the type of hypoglycemic drug you are taking.

If taking magnesium, do not take it within 2 hours of taking any kind of drug. If you have severe kidney or heart disease, you need to avoid magnesium and consult with your doctor on its use.

Magnesium is considered safe for pregnant women.

Foods High in Magnesium
hlorophyll is high in magnesium and chlorophyll comes in capsules. These are some of the foods that are high in magnesium.
Greens, berries, wheat germ, grains, nuts, cornmeal, apples, apricots, oats, pears, pecans, spinach, tofu, lentils, honey, fish, cabbage, avocados, cashews, peas, prunes, soy milk, chard

Method 38: Mineral – Iron

Excessive use of iron supplements can cause constipation. To avoid constipation, you should only use between 18 – 30 mg of iron.

Foods that contain iron are:

Dulse, rice bran, agar, almonds, black cherries, greens, lentils, dried fruits, pinto beans, raisins, rye, sesame seeds, spinach, wheat bran, liquid chlorophyll.

Kelp

Kelp should be taken daily. This provides you with a wide variety of minerals, so necessary to rebuild your colon, but also to regain good colon function.

Manganese

Manganese works with the B vitamins to strengthen the nerves. It is the nerves in your colon walls that help to activate peristaltic action.

Foods high in manganese are: Black walnuts, celery, greens, mint, oats, parsley, pineapple, watercress, apples, almonds, beans, blueberries

Health Tip: Pregnant women should not take more than 5 mg of manganese each day.

Health Drug Alert: Absorption of manganese is decreased when using antacids or anti-ulcer drugs.

Recommend manganese dose is 5 – 15 mg daily, taken with meals.

Method 39: Potassium and Prunes

Potassium is needed in your colon walls to insure that peristaltic action occurs. Without potassium, colon walls are weak and unable to respond and contract properly, when fecal matter needs to be move.
Potassium in your colon wall tissues brings in more oxygen, which is required for good cell function. In addition, potassium creates an alkaline environment inside and outside the cell, which help protect cell walls from germs.

Potassium is a powerful source, when it comes to cleaning, feeding, and building your colon walls. Removing the thin layer of buildup – harden mucus, dried fecal matter, waste derby, heavy metals - against your colon walls can be accomplished by eating those foods that are high in potassium.

Excess buildup on your colon walls of fecal matter and toxins is a cause of continual constipation. This build up prevents your colon walls from functioning properly.

Potassium is also necessary for reducing anxiety and depression. These conditions can affect peristaltic movements of your colon. Lack of it causes muscles and organs to sag and lack tone.

Potassium, also, draws water out of the body. So when potassium is in your colon it attracts water and pulls it into the fecal matter.

To add more potassium to your diet, make the following drink.

Pouring hot water over dried prunes and waiting 10 minutes. Then eat the prunes and drink the juice. Or, make a prune smoothie as shown in the Smoothie chapter. Do this on an empty stomach in the morning.

The high concentration of potassium and vitamin A, in prunes, stimulates enzymatic processes. These processes melt down fecal wall wastes and dissolve blockages. They activate peristaltic action, to move this waste out your rectum.

The foods that are high in potassium are:

Avocados, apricots, Kale, cabbage, yellow tomatoes, spinach, carrots, broccoli, cucumbers, cauliflower, alfalfa sprouts, goat milk, sesame seeds, wheat germ brewer's yeast, flax seed, grapes, green peppers, pineapples, beets, potatoes with skin, cantaloupes, raisins, broccoli, pinto beans, bananas, sweet potatoes, Blackstrap molasses

Health Alert: If you have any kidney disease, do not take potassium supplements, unless directed by your doctor. If you are pregnant, take potassium only under a doctor's direction.

Health Drug Alert: If you are on any type of drugs, do not take potassium, unless directed by your doctor.

Potassium recommended dose is 1000 – 3000 mg each day, taken with meals.

Silicon

Silicon is necessary to firm up and strengthen all the wall structures in your body - blood vessels, colon walls, organ walls, and lymph walls. It is necessary for nerve impulses to move smoothly from the brain to the vital organs and body.

When you have lost tone in your colon, by using laxatives or continual constipation, add silicon to your diet.

One of the highest foods in silicon is rice bran syrup or rice polishing. Other foods to consider are:

Oats, barley, kelp, cabbage, apricots, asparagus, beans, nectarines, plums, onions, tomatoes, seeds, nuts, wheat germ, wheat bran, raisins, pumpkin, apples, beets, brown rice, whole wheat, turnips, raisins, green beans

Recommend dose for silicon is 5 – 20 mg each day with meals.

Sodium

Organic sodium, not table salt, is necessary for a number of body functions, including your colon. Organic sodium is obtained by eating fruits, vegetables, seeds, nuts, grains, and legumes. Sodium is also found in dairy foods, meat, and fish.

The Liver and gallbladder need sodium, so that the liver does not become enlarged and the gallbladder does not produce gallstone. In your colon, sodium helps to reduce mucus formation and helps to preserve the proper pH for the good bacteria to flourish. In your joints, sodium keeps them flexible.

In the blood and lymph liquid, sodium keeps calcium in solution. Without sufficient sodium, calcium precipitins and forms bone spurs. It causes calcium to deposit in joints causing arthritic pain.

Without sodium, your body would become acidic and attract all kinds of pathogen, which create deadly diseases. Sodium helps to control and neutralize body acids and can keep your body alkaline.

An alkaline body is what you need to work towards, because diseases do not like an alkaline environment. Most people have an acid body, since they lack organic sodium and other alkalizing minerals.

You can get organic sodium from,

Cow or goat whey, black figs, kale, lentils, okra, black olives, Barley, cabbage, carrots, celery, parsley, prunes, sesame seeds, Chickpeas, cheeses, asparagus, beets, coconuts, dates, dulse.

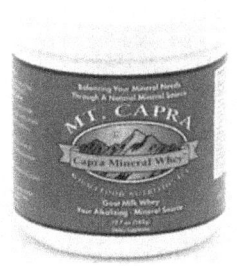

One of the best supplements for organic sodium and other electrolyte minerals is a product called, Whex or Capra Mineral Whey.

Method 39: Blackstrap Molasses

Blackstrap molasses is a strong laxative. It is

the residue that occurs after sugar cane is processed. Because sugar cane roots go deep into the ground, it contains high levels of minerals. These minerals remain in blackstrap molasses, and the sugar is left with practically none.

Blackstrap is high in potassium, calcium, and phosphorous minerals. It also contains some iron, copper, magnesium and B- vitamins.

You can add a teaspoon or tablespoon to your juices or smoothies on occasion.

Add 1 to 2 tablespoons of molasses a day to hot cereal or mix with warm water and drink it.

Honey

Honey has a large quantity of phenolics, which have antioxidant properties. These phenolics tie up free radicals and prevent damage to arteries throughout your body.

Honey has mild laxative properties. Start by taking a tablespoon three times a day. Add honey to your food, water, drinks or smoothies. Use it the way you like to eat it, but use only for a limited time, since it is like sugar.

12: Nut and Seed Constipation Remedies

Nuts and seeds contain minerals, vitamins, and oils. They can be grounded, chopped, and left whole. In grounded up form, they can be eaten with cereal, fruit, or salads. Or, if you prefer you can eat them whole, as a snack.

Nuts and seeds contain a lot of fiber and oils that help to keep you regular and help to relieve your constipation.

Method 40: Flax Seeds

Freshly ground flaxseeds help to soften stools. Take 1 tablespoon of flax seeds three times a day. (One tablespoon of flax seeds is equal to 1.5 grams of plant omega-3 fatty acid.) For severe constipation, take two tablespoons of flax seeds three times a day. These seeds can be taken whole or ground up in a coffee grinder.

Health Tip: Grind the seeds and use them immediately to get the benefit of fresh seeds and to avoid their oxidation. Your stomach will not dissolve the whole seed, but they will bulk up. Grind them open and you get the benefit from the oils and nutrients that are inside.

You can eat whole flax seeds, but you need to chew them well to break them up. Your stomach will not dissolve whole flax seeds. Chew about a tablespoon in the morning. Then drink 8 oz. of water.

You can grind them up in a grinder and add them to your salads, yogurt, morning cereal, cottage cheese, and smoothies. It is best not to use them in any cooking recipes. Heat destroys the nutritional value of the flax oil and makes them toxic.

I don't recommend you buy grounded flax seeds. You can use flax seeds in your drinks or food soon after grinding so they don't lose their nutritive value.

Flax seeds are composed of,

41% fat – fifty seven % is omega 3

18 % is monounsaturated

16% is omega 6

9% is saturated.

20% is protein

7% is moisture

It is the high level of omega 3 in flax seeds that makes them an essential seed to use in your diet. Flax seed oil helps to decrease the bad effects of omega 6, found high in olive oil. When you eat too much omega 6, you create chronic diseases.

Health Alert: In pregnant women, omega 6 in olive oil blocks the transfer of omega 3 to the baby. This is why a diet should consist of two to three parts omega - 6 and one part omega 3.

Method 41: Walnuts and Almonds

Grind equal parts of walnuts and almonds in a coffee grinder. Mix them with dark honey into a small ball. Eat this 3 times a day, with two tablespoons of warm water.

Method 42: Flax Seeds, Seeds, and Nuts

Mix equal parts of flax seeds, almonds, sunflower seeds and sesame seeds. It is o.k. to mix only three of these seeds, if that is all you have.

Grind them in a coffee grinder to a power. You can eat the power or add it to a nondairy smoothie, a juice, or morning cereal. You can also sprinkle it on your evening salad. Use up to three tablespoons twice a day.

This mixture will provide you with extra fiber, a batch of minerals, and a variety of good oils

Health alert: Drink plenty of water, when using ground up seeds.

Flax seeds are astringent and have laxative action. They are good for mild or moderate symptoms of constipation.

Health alert: Using an excess of flax seeds, can contribute to constipation. Flax seeds also have small traces of prussic acid, which is toxic in large amounts. But, it would take a lot of flax seeds to reach the toxic level.

Place between 1 teaspoon to 1 tablespoon of flax seeds in 8 oz. of warm water and let it sit for one hour. Then, just before going to bed, drink the 8 oz. After drinking this glass of flax seeds, drink another 4-8oz of water.

Method 43: Flax Seeds and Apple Cider Vinegar

Boil 1 ½ cups of distilled water.

Add 1 tablespoon of flax seeds and continue boiling the water for 10 minutes. This mixture will become jelly like. After this cools down, add 1 teaspoon of apple cider vinegar. Drink cup of this combination in the morning and until you get good daily bowel movement.

Apple cider vinegar (ACV) is another extremely important food you should include in your daily eating. ACV is high in various minerals and in particular, potassium.

Method 44: Flax seeds and oat bran

To get your bowels moving again, prepare the following mixture.

Mix 1 tablespoon of flax seeds and one tablespoon of oat bran into a glass of distilled water. Let it sit overnight. First thing in the morning, take two tablespoons. Wait half an hour, before eating anything. Do this every morning, until your bowels start moving.

Method 45: Flax Seed Oil

Our body does not make omega - 3 oil, and we need to get it from our diet.

For constipation, mix one tablespoon of flax seed oil with goat or plain cow yogurt. Add a little honey, if you like. Take this mixture right about ½ hour before bedtime.

Health Alert: Do not heat flax seed oil and keep it refrigerated. Heating it may cause some cancer-causing compounds.

Method 46: Fenugreek Seeds

Use 1-2 teaspoons of fenugreek seeds with juice or water, 2-3 times each day.

This seed will bulk up like psyllium seeds, so drink plenty of water during the day.

Health Drug Alert: Fenugreek can lower blood sugar levels, so check with your doctor before using it with diabetic drugs. Pregnant women should not use fenugreek, because of its ability to stimulate contractions.

Psyllium, Flax, Fenugreek Seed Combination

Combine flax seeds, fenugreek seeds, and Psyllium seeds. Use 3 tablespoons of this combination each day. Place them in a glass of water and drink. Make sure you drink plenty of water, during the day to help push these seeds through your colon.

Pumpkin seeds

Pumpkin seeds are a mild laxative, which can activate peristalsis. Eat seeds that are still in the shell throughout the day. You can also grind them up and add them to your salads or smoothies. If you have parasites, these seeds will help you get rid of them.

Method 47: Black Sesame Seeds

For chronic constipation, Maoshing Ni, Ph.D., C.A. and Cathy McNease, B.S., M.H., in their book, The TAO of Nutrition, 1987, recommended using black sesame seeds.

Grind black sesame seeds into a meal, by using a small coffee grinder. Mix with dark honey into a small ball.

Eat one three times a day dipped in rice wine.

Black sesame seeds also provide nutrition and action on the liver, intestines, kidney, and blood.

You can also prepare a sesame seeds soup with brown rice.

- Soak 10 parts of sesame seeds with 1 part brown rice in distilled water.

- After they are soft, about an hour, pour out the water grind them in a small food grinder to produce liquid. Strain the remaining liquid to remove coarse particles.

- Dilute this liquid with distilled water and add some honey.

- Cook on low heat until liquid becomes syrupy. Drink around two cups, within hour or so, to relieve constipation.

Method 48: Sunflower seeds

Sunflower seeds promote regularity. Use them raw shelled and unsalted every day. They contain omega-6 fatty acid just like olive oil. You can use them grounded and add them to your morning smoothie, 1-2 teaspoons, or to your homemade salad dressing.

- Add them to your salad

- Add them to your morning cereal

Here's a sunflower drink you can make.

- Take 1-2 tablespoons of sunflower seeds.

- Grind them in a coffee grinder.

- Add them to a cup of boiling water.

- Sweeten this mixture with honey, maple syrup, or blackstrap molasses.

Drink this combination morning and night to help your with you constipation.

Method 49: Coconuts

Coconuts can relieve your constipation. Eat fresh coconut two-time a day, once in the morning and in the evening.

Coconuts are high in saturated fat, which is not bad for you, since it is a short-chain fatty acid. But saturated fat, which is a long-chain fatty acid, is not good for you in large quantities. It is this fat in coconuts that allowing fecal matter to flow smoothly through your colon.

13: The Truth about Fiber and Constipation

What is Fiber?

Fiber is a carbohydrate that comes from the cell walls and structure of plants, grains, legumes, fruits, and vegetables. Most processed or junk food has little fiber, which was removed during processing.

Most people eat around 7-12 grams of fiber each day. You should be eating from 25 – 35 grams each day, to prevent serious illnesses in your body.

A diet with 40 grams of fiber provides plenty of protection and prevention against diseases, such as kidney stones, varicose veins, obesity, heart disease, appendicitis, colon disease, diabetes, appendicitis, diverticulosis, and many others. However, eating 40 grams of fiber each day, can be difficult.

When you eat fiber, it passes into your colon without getting digested in the small intestine. The good bacteria will use some of it as food, which makes them stronger and able to multiply.

Eating fiber reduces your fecal matter transit time from 3 days to 1 1/ 2 - 2days.

All processed foods, such as white flour products, have little or no fiber. Fiber is removed when various natural flours or grains are processed to make junk food. During this processing, nutrients, vitamins, and minerals are also removed.

Only plant foods and lightly processed grains have fiber of varying amounts. Foods that are "fortified" with vitamins and minerals are unbalanced, since manufacturers cannot replace all the nutrients the food once had.

Fiber, bulk, or roughage is one of the main nutrients you need to eat daily to relieve and prevent constipation and to prevent many other diseases. Fiber is a non-digestible, complex carbohydrate. Most fiber is fermented in your colon and provides some energy for the body. Fiber has two forms – soluble and insoluble.

Soluble Fiber

Soluble Fiber becomes gummy and viscous after it dissolves in water.

Soluble fiber can slow down digestion in the small intestine and prevent simple sugars from entering your bloodstream right away.

Because, it absorbs water, soluble fiber softens and gives weight to fecal matter. This makes fecal matter easier to pass through your colon.

Soluble fiber consists of pectin, gum, and mucilage. Pectin is found in carrots, apples, beets, cabbage, citrus fruits, and bananas. Gums and mucilage are found in oat bran, sesame seeds, oats, oatmeal, legumes, guar gum, and gum Arabic.

Besides helping prevent constipation, soluble fiber provides the following benefits.

- reduces the risk of heart disease

- reduces the risk of gallstones

- helps to remove toxic heavy metals and toxins from your colon

- helps to prevent the toxic condition call appendicitis
- regulates movement of sugar into the bloodstream
- helps to prevent hemorrhoids and fissures
- lowers cholesterol
- lowers absorption of fats in the intestines
- and most importantly, helps prevent the overgrowth of bad bacteria in your colon.

Insoluble Fiber

Insoluble fiber does not dissolve in water and consists of cellulose, hemi cellulose, and lignin. This type of fiber is extremely beneficial for your health. Because your body's enzymes cannot break down this fiber, like it does food, it remains in tack, as it travels through your intestines and colon.

Insoluble fiber helps fecal matter travel faster through the small intestine and your colon.

It provides bulk to your fecal matter. It makes your stools larger, softer, and stimulates peristaltic movement, as it touches your colon walls.

Insoluble fiber, like soluble fiber, slows down digestion. It also slows down absorption of protein, starch and fat and can inhibit the action of digestive enzymes.

Insoluble fibers are found in vegetables, wheat, and wheat bran. This type of fiber is considered an anti-carcinogen and a digestive aid. It is credited with preventing colon cancer and many other colon diseases.

Cellulose – Insoluble Fiber

Cellulose is a non-digestible carbohydrate, which is found on the skins of fruits and vegetables – peas, green beans, carrots, broccoli, beets, brazil nuts, and lima beans. Cellulose helps to remove cancer-causing toxins from your colon walls. It helps to prevent constipation, colitis, varicose veins, and hemorrhoids.

Hemi-cellulose is found in cabbage, peppers, green vegetables, and beets. The benefits of this fiber are:

- absorbs water in your colon and makes your stools softer

- aids in weight loss

- prevents constipation

How much bran should you take for good bowel regularity? Each person is different. You need to experiment. Start with two teaspoon each day and work towards 10 teaspoons a day or until you have bowel movements without effort or straining.

There are four basic bran products – wheat, corn, oat, and rice. They all provide a solid source of fiber in varying amounts. Make sure the bran you use is 100% unprocessed bran.

Use bran for a few weeks, to get your bowel movements back to normal. Eating bran should get your bowels moving, in a few days or less.

Once your bowels are back to normal, back off from using a lot of bran and depend more on fiber from eating more fruits, vegetables, nuts, and seeds.

There are many new food products and cereals, which use added bran. Although these products can be useful, use them for a limit time.

Wheat Bran

Many people use wheat bran, to get more fiber in their diet. This was something that was encouraged in the past. But now, you should limit or reduce the use of wheat bran as a way to get more fiber in your diet.

Wheat bran is not the best bran to use, but can be used in combination with oat, rice, or corn bran, which is better.

Wheat bran consists mainly of insoluble fiber. It consists of cellulose, hemi-cellulose, lignin, pectin, and pentosans. It absorbs plenty of water, making your stools bulky and soft, which allows them to move through your colon easily. Bulky fiber stools help to scrub your colon walls to keep them clean of mucus and toxic build up.

There are many more nutritious ways to add fiber to your diet.

Eating any bran requires drinking plenty of water throughout the day, otherwise it can cause constipation.

Health Alert: When eating bran in any form, cereal, pancakes, or muffins, always drink extra water during the day. Bran absorbs water and becomes larger. Use water to help move it easily through your colon.

Young children should not eat wheat or rice bran. Eating bran requires drinking plenty of water throughout the day. Eating too much bran can cause your fecal matter to become too bulky and can cause constipation instead of relieving it.

Bran contains a high level of phytates, which interferes with absorption of calcium, zinc, iron and copper. For this reason, use a maximum of 1/3 of a cup of bran each day for yourself. For your children use 1/6 of a cup. Excess use of wheat bran would require taking calcium, zinc, iron and copper supplements.

Bran is also high in B-vitamins and consists of around 21% protein.

Children should not eat as much fiber as adults. Children should eat oat cereals, whole grain cereals, fruits and vegetables.

Corn Bran

Corn bran has even more fiber than wheat bran by 40%. So, corn bran is excellent for prevent constipation. Both corn bran and wheat bran should be used in moderation and not used as the main ingredient in trying to prevent constipation. Most corn is now a genetically modified organism, GMO. This makes corn bran not as desirable as the other bran.

Oat Bran

Oat bran has both soluble and insoluble fiber, which make its better to use than wheat bran. However, it does have less insoluble fiber than wheat and rice bran. It can be found with relatively little processing, which helps to maintain its high quality of protein, carbohydrates and vitamins.

Health Tip: Keep away of commercially made oat, wheat or other type of bran muffins or baked products, since they contain a lot of fat, sugar and other additives that are unhealthy for you.

Rice Bran
For preventing constipation, rice bran is better than wheat bran.

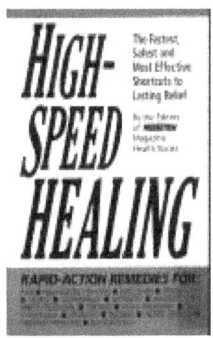

In their book called High Speed Healing, 1991, the editor of Prevention Magazine Health Books, said that, "You may see a dramatic improvement in your fight against constipation by using rice bran- instead of wheat – to increase the size and frequency of your stools. One European study says that rice beats the living chaff out off wheat when it comes to fecal output and frequency of bowel movements."

Health Tip: Do not take your calcium supplement with bran cereals, since fiber can interfere with calcium absorption.

Do not use cereal with bran in it. This bran has been processed and has lost some of its fiber content. Use the bran sold as coarse granules. Add it to your morning cereals, smoothies, shakes, cottage cheese, yogurt, or other dishes.

In his book, Inner Cleansing, 1983, Carlson Wade recommends what he calls, "Morning Bran Booster Tonic" Cleansing Rewards:

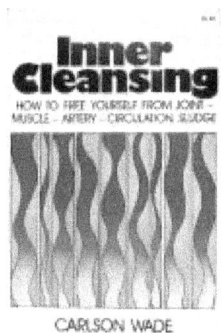

The pure bran fiber is propelled by enzymes in the juice, to scour and cleanse your digestive system in the morning. Your cells become washed and are now able to be renewed through the collagen-forming action of "In a glass of fresh vegetable juice, add two tablespoons of non-processed whole grain bran. Add a squeeze of lemon or lime juice for a piquant flavor. Blenderize for just 20 seconds and drink slowly right after your breakfast. Vitamin C from fruits you eat later on. You will experience an inner cleansing and cellular rejuvenation that will make you feel younger than young!"

Soy Bran

Soy bran is not a recommend source of bran. Despite the popularity of soy, there are some effects of soy that are not healthy. Soy is a high source of lignin fiber and other chemicals, which can block absorption of:

- minerals
- protein
- trypsin

Soy also has a high-level of phytoestrogens, which help to reduce the harmful effects of excess estrogen but soy products are not good for children who do not need a high-level phytoestrogens.

Soy used fermented – miso or tempeh –is an excellent food but still have traces of chemicals that block the body's absorption of certain minerals. Tofu can be used but should be eaten with foods high in minerals.

Despite the efforts of the soy industry to remove some of the chemicals that are not good for human consumption, there are still traces of these chemicals in soymilk and tofu.

Most soy beans grown are now considered GMO products.
Sources of Insoluble Fiber

- Bananas

- Broccoli

- Brown rice

- Brussels sprouts

- Cauliflower

- Cabbage

- Corn

- Lentils

- Potatoes

- Spinach wheat germ

- Whole wheat bread

- Whole wheat crackers

Sources of Soluble Fiber

Oranges, grapefruit, nectarines, peaches, tangerines, apples, berries, apricots, bananas, figs, prunes

Zucchini, turnips, okra, cabbage, peas, sweet potatoes
Carrots, celery, broccoli, cauliflower, corn, eggplant, okra,
Zucchini, greens
Barley, chickpeas, split peas, pinto beans, kidney beans, navy beans, potatoes

Health Alert: If you have a colon disease, check with your doctor, before including more fiber in your diet.

Remember each one of us needs a different amount of fiber. You decide how much fiber you should include in your diet. Just make sure it is more than 30 gm. each day.

Health Tip: If you are pregnant or lactating eating fiber is considered safe.

14: Constipation Remedies that can Help You

Method 50: Hot and Cold Water Jet

You can get relief from constipation, using a hot and cold "jet water shower." Here's how to do it.

Turn the water on in your morning shower. Turn your showerhead, so it has a small circular spray pattern. Change the water temperature to be as hot as you can stand it. Point the spray to your abdominal area and twist your body, right to left then left to right, until you cover the entire area.

Now, reduce the hot water, and turn on the cold water just to the point you can stand. Twist your body again, so the water covers your abdomen area.

Repeat this hot-cold sequence around seven times. At first, you might start with only a few times, until you get used to the hot, then abrupt cold shower water.

Applying hot-cold water in this fashion, stimulates the blood in your intestinal area. Additional blood to this area helps to remove toxins from your colon and to bring nutrients to reestablish your colon function.

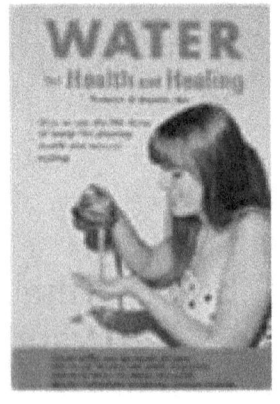 In his book, Water for Health and Healing, Federick M. Rossiter, M.D. points out, "There is no therapeutic measure in all medical science which is capable of producing more powerful general stimulation of all the functions for the body, beneficially, than a scientific application of water to the skin: cold water, alternating hot-cold-hot, and particularly the "jet health spray"'

Method 51: Body Massage

Massage of the abdominal area is a great way to tone the muscles in your colon area, provided this is done regularly. If you are trying to relieve constipation, then you can massage for a week or two, until you get past your constipation. Regular massaging can be of great benefit to your health.

You can do the massage with oils, as you lie in your bed, or in the shower, where you can use a soap solution to slide your hand over your abdomen with relative easy.

Start on the right side down near your appendix. Start with small circular or short up-down movements, and move upward toward your rib cage. This is the direction your fecal matter travels, in your colon. If you have long fingernails, you may have a problem doing this massage.

When you start your circular massage near your appendix, you are also strengthening your ileocecal valve. In the shower, massage this spot to strengthen and tone your ileocecal valve.

This valve is the gateway between your small intestine and your colon. You want a strong valve at this point, so once fecal matter moves into your colon and it will not go backward into your small intestine.

Health Tip: Massage your ileocecal value every day in the shower or with oil just before getting out of bed for 1-minute or so.

Now, once you've reached the rib cage, move to the left to the outer point of the left rib cage. Now move downward a good length toward your groin.

As you massage, notice if you find areas that have a slight pain or a lot of pain. With areas that have a slight pain, you can probably reduce the pain with daily massages.

Health Alert: With areas of deep pain, do not continue the massage. Consider consulting with a doctor, if the pain persists.

These massages will help to loosen and move fecal matter that is stagnant in your colon. Combine this massage with other constipation clearing methods listed here and that should help to clear your constipation.

Method 52: Massage on the Toilet

When you are on the toilet, there are four things you can do to help have a bowel movement, without straining.

- Add a small stool, so when you sit on the toilet your feet are raised slightly. Without a stool, bring you head down, between your legs. At this point you can also rock side to side to help move your fecal matter.
- Sit up straight and raise your arms straight up in the air.
- Sit up straight and rock sideways, from left to right, to stretch your descending colon and sigmoid. You will find that as you rock to the left or right your fecal matter will start to move.
- Sit up straight, raise your chest, and start moving your belly inward and outward. This moves your colon back and forth and helps to move your fecal matter.

These positions and movements will reduce the amount of straining you do, while having a bowel movement. These methods are helpful, until you get control of your constipation.

Anus - rectum massage

When you are sitting or standing, tighten and relax your anus area in cycles. This contracting exercises the muscles in the rectum area and stimulates the glands in this area to secrete natural lubrication. This helps to move hard stools out of your rectum and also flushes out stale blood in your anus, to help prevent hemorrhoids

Method 53: Herb Massage Oil

Make a massage oil of black pepper, marjoram and rosemary. Add one drop of each oil in a lite carrier oil like olive, almond, or sesame. Rub this mixture into your abdominal area, just before bedtime and just after your morning shower.

Castor Oil

Apply 3 – 4 drops of lukewarm castor oil, over your navel at night. This stimulates you to have a bowel movement in the morning.

Method 54: Digestive Enzymes

Health Alert: Be carefully when using HCL supplements. If your stomach is normal, additional acid can cause stomach ulcers or irritate your stomach lining.

Digestion and assimilation of food start in the mouth. As your food travels into your stomach, Hydrochloric Acid, HCL, works on the protein, and in your small intestine, digestive enzymes complete the breakdown of your food.

Your stomach produces HCL, whenever you eat protein, fat, or are stressed. When you overeat or eat too frequently, your stomach cannot produce enough HCL to digest the protein or fat you have eaten. This results in incomplete protein digestion, bloating, or gas.

Secreting good levels of HCL, stimulates the pancreas to release adequate levels of digestive enzymes.

Method 55: Barley

Eating muffins or other breads made from barley flakes or flour has shown to clear up constipation. Eat around 3 muffins each day. Make sure you drink plenty of water, during the day. Barley has been found to reduce heart, cancer, and digestive problems

Method 56: Beans

All kinds of bean and peas can help erase your constipation and prevent it. Beans have are high in fiber and will make your stools softer and increase their size. Beans also stimulate the good bacteria in your colon, by providing short chain fatty acids, which they use for food. **Here's how to use beans for constipation.**

Cooking - Clean beans with distilled water to remove dirt and small rocks. Do this three times. Soak beans for 4-8 hours. Dump water and place beans into a crock-pot. Set the pot to low and add some garlic cloves, onions, and chili power. Add other seasonings that you like.

At the low setting, the beans will cook under 112 deg F. At this temperature the enzymes in the beans will not be destroyed. These cooked beans will be considered live food. Cook the beans for around 8 hours or until soft and eatable. Eat one half cup to one cup of beans daily to break up constipation.

Here is a list of the fiber in one cup of different types of beans:

- Black eye beans 7.4 grams

- peas, canned 5.4 grams

- Kidney beans 5.0 grams

- Pinto beans 4.6 grams

- Navy beans 4.6 grams

- Lentils 1.7 grams

A Lentils Soup Remedy

Here a soup recipe that will relieve your constipation.
- Cook lentils and make a soup

- Add cooked brown rice

- Add carrots, celery, onions, and garlic

- Add a tablespoon of lecithin when adding the carrots

After the soup is make and starts to cool, add tablespoon of flaxseed oil

Method 557: Prune Juice, Applesauce, and Oat Bran

Mix, in a bowl, equal amounts of,

- Prune juice
- Applesauce
- Oat bran or any other bran
- Six ground up almond
- A squeeze of lemon

Make the consistency to your liking. Take 3 tablespoons or more each day. Best time is morning, noon and night.

Method 58: Agar-Agar

Agar is a type of seaweed that can be used to help relieve constipation in 2-8 day, if you use it every day. Boil it in water to dissolve it, then poor it into a bowel to form a jelly. Flavor it with a juice, a fruit puree, and honey or any other type of flavoring that appeal to you. Then let it to cool at room temperature until it sets.

Method 59: Sea Salt Drink

Saltwater has a fast action, in clearing out your colon. If you need to clear your constipation fast, this is the method to use. Do not use this method often, since it purges everything out of your colon, good or bad. After using this method, follow it with a week or two of good bacteria supplements.

Salt has a softening effect on hard fecal matter in your colon and helps to lubricate your colon walls. Limit your salt intake, if you have high blood pressure or edema. Salt, in excess, has a damaging effect on your blood. However, seaweeds, herbs, vegetables that contain sodium and other mineral salts are not harmful to the body.

It is best to use sea salt, for this cleansing. Sea salt has many minerals that are beneficial to your health. Only use regular salt, if cannot get sea salt.

Add two teaspoons of sea salt to a glass of warm distilled water. Drink on an empty stomach. Drink first thing in the morning. You should have a bowel movement, within one hour.

Health Alert: Do not use this method if you have edema or hypertension

Bentonite

Bentonite is a natural clay mineral that comes from volcanic ash that has eventually become clay. This clay has special properties that enable it to clean out your colon of toxic matter. It is high in sodium and this gives it electrical properties that help bind toxic matter to its atomic structure.

Bentonite is useful in assisting fruits and vegetables to clean out your colon and make it an area more livable for good bacteria. It also is good for reducing constipation.

Choose only high purity bentonite, which contains high levels of sodium and low levels of calcium. **Great Plains Bentonite** makes one such product.

Reflexology

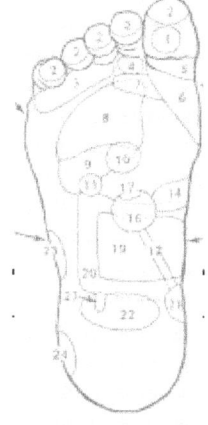

For some people, using reflexology can relieve constipation. This can be done by your own massage at the bottom of your feet and the web part of your hand between the thumb and the index finger.

The part to massage is the center portion of the bottom of your foot or the arch. To increase the pressure in this area, you can roll your foot over a golf ball. Or, you can simply massage your entire arch, especially near the heel,(#19,and #20) with your thumb, for 10 to 15 minutes. Of course, you can ask your partner to massage this area for you.

As Laura Lee Ostrowski, Reflexologist says, "Constipation can, in fact, be relieved for many people, with reflexology. I've had numerous clients see me with this complaint and had relief after receiving Reflexology. I've had some clients come for other complaints and found relief from their constipation as a bonus."

15: Devastating Illnesses Caused by Constipation

In this chapter, we will cover the symptoms, conditions, and illnesses that are associated with constipation.

Perhaps the most critical thing to understand about constipation, whether it happens only once in a while or frequently year after year is that:

Fecal matter that stays in your colon longer than it should forms a toxic bundle. This bundle then becomes the source for a toxic colon and body. A toxic colon and body set the stage, for various illnesses that can make your life miserable or can shorten your life.

When you have constipation, you have fecal matter in your colon that needs to come out. Fecal matter that stays too long in your colon hardens, decays, and becomes putrefied.

In their book, Encyclopedia of Natural

Medicine, 1991, Michael Murray, N.D. and

Joseph Pizzorono, N.D, points out that,

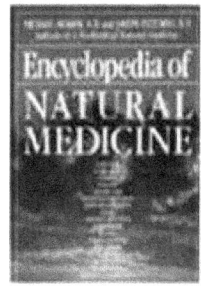

"Antigens and toxins from bowel bacteria have been found to be possibly related with the development of diabetes mellitus, meningitis, myasthenia gravis, thyroid disease, ulcerative colitis, and other diseases."

When you are constipated you will have various symptoms you may not associate with your condition. You could have a feeling of being-out-of-sorts or being depressed. You could have headaches, bad breathe, sour stomach, bloating, abdominal pain and hardness.

What are some of the symptoms or conditions that are caused by constipation?

This list is long.

- Abdominal discomfort, gas pain, heartburn

- Acid Reflux
- Alternating constipation – diarrhea
- Appendicitis
- Arthritis
- Back Pain
- Ballooned colon
- Boils, Pimples, and Skin Rashes
- Breast Cancer
- Cellulite
- Colitis
- Colon cancer
- Colon Degradation
- Diverticulosis
- Excessive bad bacteria
- Flatulence
- Growth of unfriendly bacteria – bad bacteria use decayed

- fecal matter and create by products that cause cancer and
- other illnesses
- Halitosis
- Headaches
- Heart problems
- Hemorrhoids
- Hernia, hiatal or inguinal hernias
- IBS
- Impaction
- Indigestion
- Insomnia
- Liver weakness
- Maldigestion
- Nagging back pains
- Nausea
- Nutritional deficiencies
- Obesity, weight gain
- Reabsorption of estrogen

- Reabsorption of bile and cholesterol

- Spastic colon

- Tight colon

- Toxic colon

- Unclear thinking

- Varicose veins

- Weight gain

- Worms, parasites

As you can see, constipation is not a simple condition to avoid. You must have daily bowel movements, so that you don't develop a toxic colon.

Acid Reflux

When fecal matter remains too long in your colon, back pressure builds up in your colon and affects the food coming into the stomach and small intestine. This pressure can cause food to be pushed backwards and gases from your colon to flow out of the mouth. This gas can irritate the throat and mouth lining and produce bad breath.

Appendicitis

The appendix is part of the lymphatic system just like tonsils. It releases lubricants and antiseptic liquids that stimulate peristalsis and protect the surrounding tissue.

Appendicitis occurs when you lack fiber in your diet. Without fiber, the fecal matter that moves into the appendix becomes stagnant and does not come out. This stagnant matter becomes putrefied and toxic and eventually leads to appendicitis.

Arthritis

Poisons from your colon can go to your joints and cause stiffness and pain. Constipation is one of the symptoms that exist, before the appearance arthritis. Continual constipation causes arthritis.

Back Pain

Back pain can be caused when you have constipation. This happens when toxins and toxic gases move from your colon into the lower-back muscles and tissues, creating weaken muscles and an acid condition.

Minerals in the lymph liquid try to neutralize all the toxic matter in your lower back tissue, but don't always succeed, especially when your body is deficient in minerals.

Continual constipation uses up much of the minerals in the lower back, creating an acid condition. These results in pain, weaken muscles, and tension that pulls the vertebrae out of position. This results in the need for a physical therapist or chiropractic care.

Adjustments the chiropractor makes will not hold, if you continue to have constipation and fail to eat foods that provide you with high levels of minerals – vegetables and fruits.

Ballooned Colon

A ballooned colon is a condition where your colon is larger than normal and expanded outward. Your colon walls have lost their strength and tone. This occurs when you are constipated, and your fecal matter remains in one spot too long. As more fecal matter accumulates in this one spot, your colon walls continue to balloon out.

Boils, Pimples, and Skin Rashes

Boils and other skin eruptions occur when your colon is overloaded with toxins. These toxins cross your colon walls and the liver routes some of them to your skin follicles. If you are constipated, the body will use your other channels of elimination to eliminate toxins from your colon – skin, kidney, lungs, and lymphatic system. These toxins, as the come into the skin, cause infections, pus, and eruptions to appear.

Breast Cancer

Constipation can also increase your risk of getting breast cancer. Constipation resulting from high levels of bad bacteria in your colon creates an environment where less bile salts and estrogen are detoxified. This condition has been related to breast cancer and cancer.

Researchers at the University of California in San Francisco have discovered that women who only have 2-3 bowel movements each week show signs of abnormal cell proliferation in the aspirated breast fluids.

In addition, toxins from a contaminated colon need to be moved out of the body. The lymphatic system helps to move and detoxify these toxins. When the body is overloaded with toxins, the lymph nodes become clogged and accumulate toxins, which prevent their removal. This condition can lead to diseases of various types.

Colitis

Colitis is an inflammatory or ulcerative condition that occurs along your colon or rectum wall.

Colitis is caused by emotional stress, excessive bad bacteria, food allergies, and poor diet. Many of the causes of colitis are similar to those that cause constipation.

Inflammation of your colon walls caused by colitis can produce bleeding, which can darken your stool color.

Health Alert: Colitis typically requires a low fiber and high-protein diet. If you have colitis, it is critical you review with a Nutritionist the type of colitis you have, so he/she can recommend the right eating plan for you.

Colon Cancer

If you have a tumor in your colon, this could block the movement of your fecal matter. This condition could cause constipation and result in small-diameter stools.
Colon cancer occurs more frequently in people who eat meat – beef or chicken. This happens because meat promotes the growth of bad bacteria. It is the bad bacteria that convert bile, from the gallbladder, into a cancer promoting substance.

Since meat typically moves slowly through your colon, cancer promoting substance have the opportunity to stay in contact with your colon walls longer and embed themselves into your colon wall.

Because fiber helps to speed fecal matter through your colon, fiber helps prevent colon cancer. In addition, fiber feeds the good bacteria, which weakening the bad bacteria and their toxic effects.

Crohn's Disease

Crohn's is a severe inflammatory condition of your colon. This inflammation typical occurs at the last portion of the small intestine, near the ileocecal valve and the start of your colon. Overtime, bowel function is affected, as it is with all other infections, inflammations, or ulcers in your colon.

Crohn's disease affects absorption of vitamin B12 and reabsorption of bile salts. Deficiencies in these nutrients can lead to other serious diseases.

Crohn's is typically caused by an infectious organism, diet, or emotional issues. Like for constipation, a high-fiber diet is recommended.

Excessive Bad Bacteria

Constipation causes bad bacteria to multiple. As fecal matter remains stagnant in your colon, the pH in your colon becomes more alkaline. Bad bacteria thrive in an alkaline condition. When your bad bacteria dominate the colon environment, your good bacteria slowly diminish.

Diverticulosis

Diverticulosis is caused by constipation. This happens when fecal matter in your colon remains too long at one spot, creating toxic weak spots along your colon walls.

Constant constipation with increased pressure from fecal matter and fecal matter gases causes these weak spots to bulge or become irritated and infected. These outward bulging spots are known as a hernia or diverticulosis.

When you have a weak or toxic point on your colon walls, the straining and the constant peristaltic action your colon makes, to move food from a poor diet, creates small pouches. These pouches can become inflamed and filled with toxic fecal matter.

As this disease becomes worse, it creates constipation, and it was constipation that created them. A high-fiber diet is recommended, if you have diverticulosis.

Flatulence

Flatulence is gas that is passed out of the rectum. This gas is created from the:

- Air we swallow during eating
- Gas created by bacteria acting on undigested food, in your colon
- Gas created by bacteria acting on fiber
- Gas created from decaying and purifying food in your colon
- Gas created in the stomach or colon because of anxiety and tension
- Gas that is contained in carbonated drinks that you drink

What kind of gas is this? Most of it is carbon dioxide with hydrogen sulfide, the smelly part of flatulence, and methane. Some ammonia gas is also created and passes through your colon walls and into the bloodstream, which then has to pass out through your urine.

When you have constipation, this gas can become trapped in your colon, creating pain and discomfort in the abdominal area.

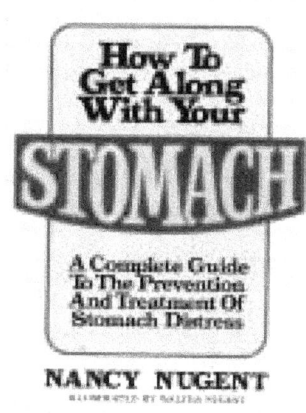

In her book, Nancy Nugent, How to get along with your Stomach, 1979, quotes Dr. Michael D. Levitt of the University of Minnesota as saying, "Ideally, the gas should then pass out through the anus as flatus, but it may become trapped

in the intestinal tract by an obstruction or by the peristaltic inactivity (constipation) cited Dr. Levitt. If so, the result will be predictable: bloating and pain."

Heart Problems

One side effect of constipation is straining to have a bowel movement. This creates an increase in blood pressure, which can trigger a heart attack in anyone with a weak heart or arteriosclerosis. This means if you have any cardiovascular conditions – high blood pressure, angina, weak arteries, and so on - you need to be careful and make sure you don't get constipated. Follow the remedies and eat the foods that are outlined throughout this book.

Hemorrhoids

Hemorrhoids are related to constipation. They are blood vessels in the lining of the rectum and anus that have enlarged. This occurs when you are constipated and have to strain and push to have a bowel movement. If you strain to have bowel movements, year after year, you will develop hemorrhoids.

Straining to have a bowel movement will also produce varicose veins, hiatal hernias, or diverticulosis.
Hemorrhoids are more common in men than women.

Hemorrhoid symptoms are bleeding, itching, mucosal discharge, protruding tissue, discomfort, and pain in the anus.

When bleeding occurs, you will see blood in your stools and it will diffuse rapidly in the toilet bowl water. If this happens, the bleeding can be stopped with natural remedies.

To give the area in the anus with hemorrhoids a chance to heal, it is necessary to have bowel movements that are free from straining and puffing. This is accomplished through the proper combination of natural laxative remedies and diet as outline in this book.

Impactions

Impactions are an accumulation of fecal matter on your colon walls. This occurs over years of eating a poor diet. This causes gummy, pasty, and sticky fecal matter, which accumulates along your colon walls.
This bowel condition is where small pockets form along your colon walls, which collect fecal matter that does not move out, during regular bowel movements. Overtime this trapped fecal matter becomes putrefied and toxic.

Impaction can also occur when fecal matter becomes attached to your colon wall where it remains despite fecal matter passing over it. It becomes harden, and later it becomes difficult to remove. Using a process call colonics can help to remove this impaction.

Liver Weakness

Constipation weakens the liver. The liver is responsible for filtering out toxins from the blood that comes from the stomach and your colon. When you have constipation, fecal matter remains longer in your colon than it should. This gives toxins the time to become absorbed into the blood and into the liver.

When the liver gets overwhelmed with toxins, the liver weakens, blood is not clean, and blood circulation is decreased. The liver produces less bile, which then affects your colon's peristaltic movement and this leads to constipation.

Estrogen Reabsorption

Constipation creates a condition where estrogen can be reabsorbed into the blood. This can lead to excess estrogen levels in the body. High estrogen levels are associated with breast cancer and infertility.

Normal bowel movements can lead to normalizing estrogen levels in the blood.

Spastic colon

Spastic colon is a condition where the walls of your colon have diminished tone and have become misshapen. When this occurs, bowel movements do not occur in a normal frequency. This condition occurs with years of poor eating habits or emotional strain.

Tight Colon

A tight occurs when excess tension exists in your colon walls. This causes the walls to narrow down and decrease the size of your colon opening. This condition leads of excessive bouts with constipation and results from anxiety and excess nervous tension. A poor diet adds to this condition.

Toxic Colon

When you have constipation, cholesterol elimination is blocked and remains in your colon, until you have a bowel movement. The longer cholesterol stays in your colon the higher chance it has of being reabsorbed into your body.

This is why fiber is necessary in your diet. Fiber helps to bind cholesterol, so it is not reabsorbed into the blood, but passed out of your colon in your stools.

Where does this cholesterol come from? It comes from the liver bile that passes into the gallbladder. The gallbladder releases this bile into the small intestine.

Fiber also binds with bile, various wastes, toxins and carcinogens in your colon, so they are not reabsorbed into your bloodstream. Without fiber, constipation occurs, allowing toxins to become fermented, decayed, and purified. These toxins can be absorbed back into your body. This condition is called a toxic colon.

Another benefit of fiber is that in your colon, fiber will delay absorption of sugar and sugary substances into the blood. This helps to prevent many other diseases related to sugar.

Unclear thinking

When your fecal matter slows down or stops moving in your colon, chances are you will experience foggy and unclear thinking. Slow moving fecal matter leads to many conditions that stress and pain your gastrointestinal system. This stress and pain partially decrease your total awareness, which reduces your clear thinking.

When you are under pain, your concentration is affected. Most of your thought is on this pain or discomfort. This is part of your survival mechanism, so that you can do something about this pain.

When you are pain free, this is the time when you will be the most creative and have the ability to have clear thinking, which can result in producing the best performance in whatever you do.

Weight Gain
When your colon becomes impacted with mucus and dried fecal matter, your colon is in a toxic state. This allows toxin to move into the body and eventually plug up the lymph nodes and lymphatic system. This blockage, as it gets more serious, can result in swelling of the legs and torso.

A toxic colon prevents the total absorption of nutrients, and this can cause you to overeat to get the nutrients your body needs.

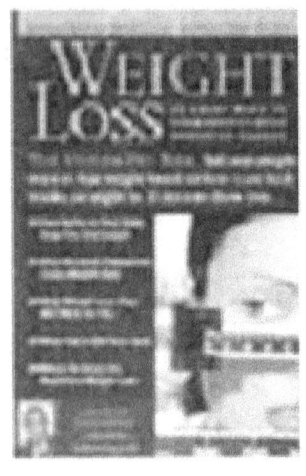

In Burton Goldberg's book, Weight Loss – Alternative Medicine Definitive Guide, 2000, Burton points out, "Toxins that build up in your colon pass through the intestinal wall and accumulate in the lymphatic system – a network of vessels and nodes that clean and drain the body of toxic substances. When the flow of toxins from your colon becomes too heavy, the lymph can become blocked and cause toxins to back up throughout the body. The result can be swelling of the torso and legs, damage to the liver and other detoxification organs and blood toxicity... this is one of the main reasons for obesity, explains naturopath Richard Anderson, N.D.,N.M.D"

Worms and Other Parasites

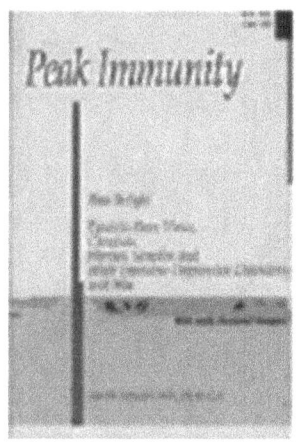 Luc De Schepper, M.D., Ph.D., C.A., in his book, Peak Immunity, reminds us that, "Millions of Americans discover each year, we have parasites too. Many, in fact, are native to this country. You can get them without leaving your home... The

parasites range in size from a microscopic single-celled protozoan to a worm that may exceed 30 feet in length."

When you have regular bowel movements, parasites don't have time to lay their eggs and this reduces the amount of parasites you will have in your colon.

16: The Cause of Constipation

Causes of constipation

Your colon is designed to move undigested matter and various bodily wastes through its tract and out the rectum. It does this naturally, but only when this matter and waste have bulk, fiber, bile, oils, water, and minerals. It is this fiber and other nutrients, which push against your colon walls that trigger peristaltic action. You can only get this healthy bulk of nutrients, when you eat plenty of fruits, vegetables, and grains that have a combination of soluble and non-soluble fiber.

Meat, fish, and dairy products have little or no fiber. In your colon, these foods do not move easily and remain too long in your colon. So, fiber and other nutrients help these foods, to move faster through your colon.

Constipation habits come from unnatural living

Constipation is a complex symptom that is caused by many conditions that have amassed in the body and caused your colon to malfunction.

Constipation can be caused by a physical weakness due to surgery, inactivity, or deformities, which were inherited or acquired through injury or surgery. Constipation cause by these conditions can be improved by using natural nutrients and alternative methods.

However, it is more difficult to help this type constipation, since the physical conditions have to be improved.

The continual use of medications or drugs of any sort can cause constipation. It can be caused by the excess use of laxatives. It can be caused continual use of certain minerals or vitamins.

Psychological constipation

Constipation is also related to psychological and emotion issues. Anxiety will cause the nerves, wall tissue and muscles in your colon to tense up. If you have a personality that holds feeling or thoughts inside you and do not discuss them with those people you should, you will mostly likely have continual constipation.

Health Alert: If you have stress and anxiety in your life, constipation can be a result. Anxiety can overwork your Adrenal gland, causing excess cortisol output. Overtime, because cortisol is toxic to the brain, cortisol will damage and kill brain cells, which can lead to premature old age and Alzheimer's. You will also feel tired and run down when you over stress your Adrenal.

Sometimes constipation can suddenly appear when changes in normal living habits and stressful conditions have occurred – flying out of your time zone, having personal confrontations at work or within your family.

Infrequent bouts with constipation are really nothing to worry about and can be corrected with many of the suggestions listed in this book.

The main cause of constipation is the continual eating of processed foods, which have little food value or fiber and are packed with poison additives. This results in colon wall weakness, where fecal matter cannot even be push out of the rectum.

Eating food with little or no fiber creates fecal matter that is mushy or hard and compacted. Mushy or compact fecal matter is hard to move along your colon and your colon walls tire after many peristaltic movements. After a time, your colon walls stop trying, and you end up with constipation.

Constipation is a body condition you have created by improper living choices, which you can change. It is sometimes an easy symptom to eliminate, and at other times it is difficult to deal with. It occurs from a complex of many things. Like so many other body conditions or illnesses, it is a result of:

- Absorbing too many toxins into your body
- Anxiety and depression
- Being bedridden
- Having colitis, or spastic colon
- Having diabetes

- Having diseases of the anus or rectum
- Having tumors, diverticulosis
- Drinking coffee
- Drinking milk
- Drinking sodas
- Drinking tea
- Eating excess protein
- Eating food that doesn't have fiber
- Eating processed foods
- Eating sugars
- Eating too much food at one sitting
- Excessive exposure to organophosphate insecticides
- Excessive use iron supplements
- Excessive use of enemas
- Excessive use of seasonings
- Excessive Calcium in the body
- Fatigue
- Food sensitivities

- High fever – colon accumulates heat and hardens stools
- Hypothyroidism - Low levels of thyroid hormone
- Kidney failure
- Lack of good bacteria
- Mineral Deficiency
- Nerve disorders of your bowel
- Not chewing food completely
- Not drinking enough water
- Not enough exercise
- Older people
- Overeating
- Overuse of laxatives
- Overdose of Vitamin D
- Parasites
- Poor digestion
- Postponing a bowel movement

- Pregnancy

- Premenstrual tension

- Spinal injuries – people with these injuries can have damage to the nerves that regulate bowel moments

- Toxic liver

- Use of prescription drugs

Health Alert: Constipation can be a symptom of the start of a disease or illness. Do not take drugstore laxatives, which will mask the illness that eventually has to be dealt with.

Absorbing too many toxins

Taking in too many toxins – pesticides, insecticides, heavy metals, food additives, and air pollution - from various sources, can create constipation. Each of these toxins and chemicals can have different reaction in your colon, which cause your colon to malfunction.

Aluminum Toxicity

Aluminum toxicity is one of those conditions you might not think much about. So, you need to be informed as to what damage excess aluminum can do and how it gets into your body.

First, aluminum in the stomach can affect digestion by binding with pepsin, which helps to break down protein.

You can get too much aluminum in your body through personal hygiene products or by using antacids. Always check the ingredients of the products you are buying for any form of aluminum.

Health Tip: If you have allergies or have had them in the past and are having reoccurring bouts with constipation, re-evaluate your allergies for new allergic substances.

High fever

When you have a fever, the heat accumulates in your colon and hardens your fecal matter. This makes it more difficult for you to have a bowel movement. When you have a fever, you should drink more water and juices.

Hypothyroidism

If you have hypothyroidism, you will experience digestive problems. You may have a loss of appetite or you may actually gain weight. Peristaltic action will decrease leading to constipation.

It is easy to check your thyroid function. Simply measure your body temperature in the morning, before you get out of bed.
As soon as you wake up, place a basal or digital thermometer into your under arm and keep still for 5 to 10 minutes. Just ignore the beeping of the digital thermometer.

Then, read the thermometer.

- Normal temperature is 97.8 F to 98.2 F

- Readings below 97.8 F indicate hypothyroidism

- Readings above 98.2 F indicate hyperthyroidism

See your doctor, if you get readings outside the normal range.
Lack of Good Bacteria

A balance between good bacteria and bad is necessary for your colon to work right. Bad bacteria are always in your colon just waiting for the opportunity to become dominant.

When your good bacteria are dominant, your risk of becoming constipated is less. Dominant good bacteria indicate your colon is working well and that fecal matter will move naturally, through your colon.

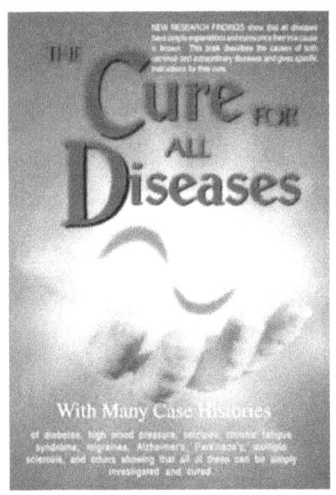

In her book, A Cure For All Diseases, 1995, Hulda Regehr Clark, PH.D, N.D., points out, "Bacteria are part of the cause; and part of the results! Constipation increases the bacteria level which causes further constipation! You may solve the constipation problem immediately by zapping. Even though this kills some "good" with some "bad" bacteria, no harm is done. The stool is re-colonized in one to two days."

Avoid using antacids, OTC laxatives, and antibiotics, since they kill good bacteria.

Mineral Deficiency

When your body is deficient in minerals, you will have an acid body that will not function well. Your colon typically recycles ionic minerals, by pulling them out of the fecal matter, moving them through your colon wall, and transferring them into your bloodstream.

You need minerals to neutralize the excess acids in your small intestine, colon and throughout your body. Without a constant supply of minerals, your colon will not function like it should.

Overeating

If you overeat, your body may not be able to digest all of this food. Undigested food is not absorbed in the small intestine and will move into your colon. This undigested food is difficult to move through your colon and can cause constipation. This slow moving undigested food will decay, create gas, and produce a toxic colon.

If you have large amounts of slow moving fecal matter in your colon, you will produce gas that can enlarge your colon. Repeated enlargement of your colon will weaken your colon walls and your peristaltic action.

Not drinking enough water

One of the functions of your colon is to remove water from fecal matter, as it passes through your colon. This prevents your body from eliminating too much water, through your stools and becoming dehydrated. The removed water is used in your blood and lymph liquid.

When you do not drink enough water, fecal matter will not move through your colon quickly. This gives your colon walls more time to remove water from your fecal matter. This in turn causes your fecal matter to become hard and dry.

When fecal matter gets hard, it becomes difficult to move through your colon. The longer it stays in your colon, the harder it gets. Peristaltic action will move it slowly, and as more fecal matter enters your colon from other meals, you will soon be constipated.

Under normal conditions, your body alerts you to when you need to drink water, by making you feel thirsty. This should be your guide to how much water to drink. The problem arises, when you ignore this thirst and your body becomes dehydrated.

This is why it is recommended you keep track of how much water you drink, 32 oz. minimum. However don't force yourself to drink more water. But do have water available, so when you feel thirsty, you can drink right away.

If you have pain in the lower left part of your abdomen because of constipation, drinking water should relieve this pain.

Not enough exercise

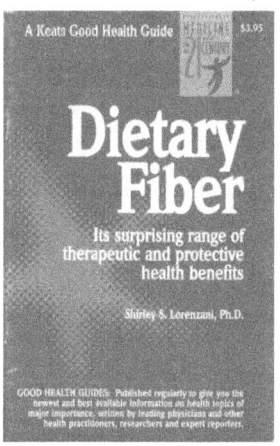

In her booklet, Dietary Fiber, 1988, Shirley S. Lorenzni, PhD, states, "Inactivity contributes to constipation. You may have noticed this during a period of bed rest or while you are traveling. Some scientists believe that lack of physical exercise, not old age, causes constipation in the elderly. A recent study in African revealed a definite connection between exercise and fecal output"

Older People

As you age, you are more likely to have constipation. As you get older, the walls of your intestines and colon weaken and lose tone. This makes it more difficult to have good strong wall movements, which are necessary to move fecal matter through your intestines and colon.

Colon weakens, when you don't supply the right minerals to your colon walls. Plenty of potassium is needed to make your colon walls flex. Potassium is obtained from both fruits and vegetables.

Colon tone is lost, when you don't exercise and eat the right foods.

Exercise forces your stomach muscles to contract and extend. This movement strengthens your intestinal and colon walls and at the same time helps to push fecal matter in your colon towards your rectum.

Cells that secrete water along the intestinal walls decrease, as you get older. Overtime, less water is secreted and absorbed by your fecal matter, making them harder. This condition makes the fecal matter more difficult to move along your colon.

Overuse of laxatives

Using laxatives, can damage nerves inside your colon walls. When used excessively, you can become dependent on them.

Drugs store laxatives can create the condition you are trying to eliminate – constipation. Use them sparingly or consult a doctor before using them. Use the natural remedies listed here for constipation and avoid using laxatives.

Parasites

Most parasites that are absorb from outside your body live in your colon. Of course, they also get into your blood, lymph liquid, organs, and skin. These parasites attach themselves to your colon walls and cause many irritating symptoms, like diarrhea, constipation, flatulence, headaches, and poor memory. They can also cause more serious problems, such as holes in your colon wall.

When this happens, fecal matter can cross your colon wall, get into your blood, and cause allergic reactions.

Don't think you don't have parasites. This would be a big mistake. Most everyone has some sort of parasites in their body.

In her book, Parasites – THE ENEMY WITHIN, Hanna Kroeger, 1991-2001, says,

"Here are some dietary suggestions. A diet high in carbohydrates and low in protein has been found to make parasitic infections worse. When the body is in an alkaline condition the parasitic infection sets in. It is best to keep the diet slightly acidic both as a preventive measure and when treating the infection. Foods that help keep the intestines acidic are apple cider vinegar and cranberry juice."

Parasite waste and excretions are toxic to your body and make your colon pH more alkaline. You need your colon to be slightly acidic. This makes your colon more livable for your good bacteria.

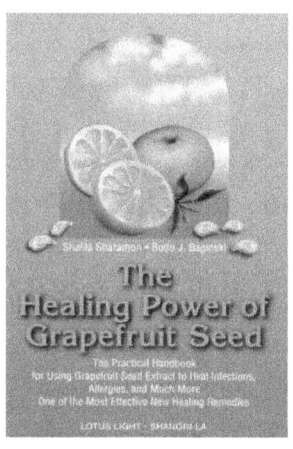

In their book, The Healing power of Grapefruit Seed, 1997, Shalila Sharamon and Bodo J. Baginski summarized the importance of using grapefruit seed extract, "After we have seen how easily pathogens -

whether they are bacteria, viruses, fungi, or parasites—get into our body and how much havoc they can wreak, the question may arise:

"Wouldn't it be smart to take a few drops of grapefruit seed extract every day as a preventative against the uninvited guests? Since it is non-toxic, it can't do any harm but will be beneficial."

How do you know if you have parasites? A few of the symptoms are:

- Bluish color in the whites of your eyes

- Itching in the rectum area

- Fingernails that are brittle, hard and are concave, curving upward

Poor digestion

Food digestion is the responsibility of many organs in your body – the mouth, stomach, liver, gallbladder, spleen, pancreas, small intestine, and colon.

When food is not broken down where it can be absorbed through the small intestine, it will continue to your colon. There in your colon, bad bacterium will break it down, causing your colon to become more alkaline. This change in pH will reduce the good bacteria population, which will eventually lead to constipation.

Postponing a bowel movement

Each time you have an urge to have a bowel movement and don't head for the bathroom, you are training yourself to be constipated. This does not happen overnight, but over many years of practice.

Delaying bowel movements can be a result of:

- Being in someone else's home
- Being where bathrooms are not readily available
- Not being able to use bathrooms, other than your own
- Only going to the bathroom, when, everything is to your satisfaction.

So here's happens when you delay the urge to go to the bathroom. When your rectum is empty, it is collapsed. From the sigmoid colon, fecal matter enters your rectum, fills it, and you get a desire to have a bowel movement. If you ignore this desire too long, the nerves in your rectum wall lose their sensitive to the fecal matter irritation and pressure.

As the fecal matter sits in your rectum, more moisture is pulled out of the fecal matter, by the rectum walls. The fecal matter becomes harder and harder the longer you delay your bowel movement. To remove this hard fecal matter, you will have to strain to push it out.

Straining and puffing to have a bowel movement will cause rectal blood vessels to enlarge and cause excessive pressure on other organs.

Postponing your bowel movement regularly will cause to become irregular.

Make sure you have your bowel movement, when the urge hits or soon after. Let other things wait, while you take care of the most important thing – a bowel movement. This is training you to maintain regular bowel movements.

Spinal injuries

People with spinal injuries can have damage to the nerves that regulate bowel moments and this result in having long-term constipation.

Pregnancy

Being pregnant can cause you to be constipated. As the fetus grows, it starts to put pressure on the stomach, intestines, and rectum. Using many of the constipation remedies given here, will help you lessen your constipation.

Toxic Liver

The liver produces bile, which is release by the gallbladder at the right time. Bile breaks up fat into small droplets, so it can be digested and absorbed in the small intestine. Bile also makes your fecal matter softer and promotes peristaltic motion.

When more fat than normal is embedded in the fecal matter, it moves slower in your colon. This is caused by fat not being completely absorbed in the small intestine
.
When the liver is toxic, it will not produce enough bile, and fat will not be properly

digested. Of course, if your gallbladder is not working well, or if it has been surgically removed, the right amount of bile will also not reach the small intestine.

Use of prescription drugs

One side of effect of some calcium channel blocker is constipation – Calan, Isoptin. Drugs like Amitril, Elavil, Endep, Janimine, Surmontil, Tofranil and Vivactil that are used to treat depression can cause constipation.

Other drugs that can cause constipation are:

Antacids

Anticonvulsants

Anticholinergics

Antihypertensives

Antidepressants

Anti-parkinsonism

Anti-psychotics

Muscle relaxants

OpiatesDiuretics

17: Prevent Constipation and Gain New Health

How do you prevent Constipation?

To prevent or relieve constipation, you need to get your bowels to move and work naturally. This means you should not be dependent on laxatives – drugstore or natural.

The natural laxatives listed in the previous chapters were to kick start your colon and move the stagnant fecal matter through your colon and out the rectum. They were for short-term use to give you quick relief from your state of constipation – one to four week or so. But, many of these techniques, with fruits and vegetables, you can incorporate into you eating habits.

When you have moved out stagnant fecal matter in your colon, you need to look closely at how to prevent constipation.

Preventing constipation will require a change in the way you eat, exercise, and think. This can sometimes be difficult. It requires a new mind-set and plenty of will power – a new lifestyle. Don't wait until you have an illness, to change your mind-set. With a lifestyle change, you can expect normal bowel movements in 2-3 weeks and 4 weeks at the latest.

Health tip: You will need a life style where you get plenty of fiber, moisture, lubrication, minerals, vitamins, nutrients, water and exercise to prevent constipation.

Older people have to be more diligent in following good eating habits than those younger. Older people's digestive abilities have slowed down and their peristaltic sensors are less sensitive.

How to Prevent Constipation

The following eating habits and lifestyles will help you prevent constipation. Don't try to make all of these changes at once. Do them gradually. Every week change one of your old eating habits. Not only will you prevent constipation, but you will be creating excellent health.

- Drink plenty of water

- Eat less processed carbohydrates
- Eat more nutritious food
- Eat plenty of fiber
- Eat the good oils
- Reduce emotional upsets – at home, office, and business
- Exercise regularly
- Feed the good bacteria
- Get plenty of rest and sleep
- Keep you colon acidic
- Take a good mineral supplement
- Use digestive enzymes

Drinking Plenty of Water

Your body needs plenty of distilled water every day to eliminate toxins from inside and outside your cells and from your blood. When you don't drink enough water, your body becomes dehydrated. This forces your body to pull water out of your fecal matter in your colon, causing constipation.

Health Tip: Drinking extra water is not only to prevent constipation; it is for preventing you from becoming dehydrated. When you become dehydrated, you are subject to many illnesses, including constipation.

If you drink more water, not all of it moves into your colon. The water you drink is absorbed through the small intestine and only a small amount will move into your colon as a lubricant and into your fecal matter.

If your body has plenty of water, it will draw less water from your colon and your fecal matter will not become dry and hard.

Best Water to Drink

What is the best water to drink? Facet water is out. There are three other forms of water to drink – regular bottled water, reverse osmosis (RO) water, and distilled water.

Distilled water is the best water to drink. It is the purest type of water and has all contaminates removed. Critics that point out this water can leach out minerals from your body. However, there is no evidence that his happens.

Reverse osmosis water is the second best water to drink.

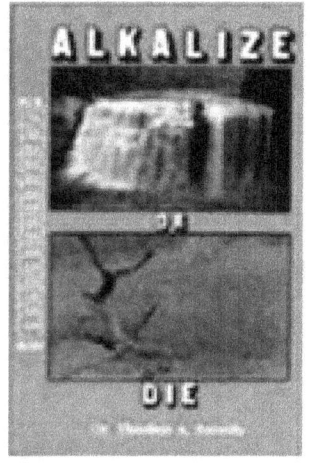 In his book, Alkalize or Die, 2002, Dr. Theodore A. Baroody, discusses distilled water. "In my opinion, distilled water and alkaline-restructured water are the safest forms of water at this time of our earth's toxic exploitation. I encounter considerable resistance to the idea of drinking distilled water. These are the myths commonly believed:

1. Distilled water leaches valuable mineral out of your body.

2. It leaches minerals out of your brain and softens it;

3. It deprives you of important minerals you need from spring water.

Why when I look for even one reputable source about the leaching out of valuable minerals from the body it is not to be found? "

Water that contains inorganic minerals is not good for you. Typically this is known as hard water. Hard water, which contains many inorganic minerals, will eventually corrode the pipes it flows through or plug them up with deposits. It will do the same in your body.

Organic minerals are different than inorganic minerals in that organic minerals are obtained from fruits and vegetables. It is organic minerals – in electrolytic form – that help to maintain life, since they combine readily with vitamins, enzymes, and other nutrients to form compounds that are usable by your body.

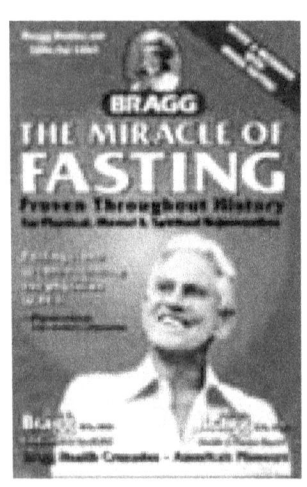

In his book, The Miracle of Fasting, Paul C. Bragg points out that, "Every liquid prescription that is compound in any drugstore the world over is prepared with distilled water. It is not true that distilled water leaches the organic minerals out of the body nor is it dead water. It is the purest and safest water that man can drink. Distilled water helps to dissolve the terrible toxic poisons that collect in people's bodies. It passes through the kidneys without leaving inorganic pebbles and stones. If you wash your hair in rain (distilled) water, you will discover the softness of natural soft water."

It is best to store distilled water in a glass container, if possible. Most plastic containers are made from polycarbonate plastic which contain Bisphenol-A. Bisphenol A has many health issues, as shown in clinical studies. When is the best time to drink water?

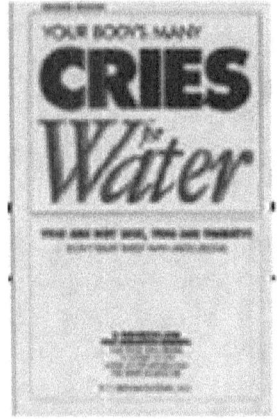

According to F. Batmanghelidj, M.D. in his book Your Body's Many Cries for Water, he says, "The best times to drink water are: One glass one half hour before taking food – breakfast, lunch, and dinner.

One glass 2 ½ hours after meals.
One glass before going to bead
One glass when you are thirsty."

Health Tip: Drink juices around 1 hour before meals.

Drink little water with your meal, since water will dilute your digestive acid, in your stomach. This will reduce your ability to digest protein. Drink water only when food accumulates in your throat.

When you do drink water with you meal, drink room temperature water and is not ice or cold water. Cold water contracts your stomach and surrounding blood vessels, stopping your digestion process.

Drink a minimum of 2 quarts of water each day. You can add a small amount of fresh juice to your water, to make it tastes better. For example, add a fresh squeezed lemon in one quart of water. Or put some fruit into your water to change it taste. If you do this, you might be able to drink more water, at least two quarts each day.

To prevent lemon acid water from etching your teeth, have another jar of water without lemon to rinse and drink from, after drinking the lemon water.

Health Tip: Add Alkalife drops to your distilled water. This product turns your water into an electrolyte –mineral water, which has minerals in ionic form. Electrolytes are the type of liquid that surrounds your cells and is capable of neutralizing acids that are harmful to your health.

What is Considered Water?

Liquids or juices that do not have added salt or sugar can be considered water. Water for your body also comes from:

- Fruit juices and fruits

- Herbal teas

- Vegetables, vegetable juices and broths

Water does not come from:
- Sodas

- Sweeten fruit juices

- Coffee with sugar

- Tea with sugar

Health Tip: Watch the color of your urine. The color should be a light yellow to colorless. If it is a dark yellow, you are not drinking enough water.

The dark yellow results from toxins and nutrients your kidney is removing from your blood. If you are not drinking enough water, toxins become concentrated and color your urine. Over time, this condition will affect the health of your kidney.

Eat less processed carbohydrates and meat

There are certain foods that have a hard time moving through your colon. These are processed foods, fried foods, meat, and dairy products. These foods contain little or no fiber, which make it difficult for you colon to push them through.

All dry foods such as bread, biscuits, bagels, crackers, bran, powdered foods, are difficult to move through your colon and can lead to constipation.

Processed foods are what cause constipation, since these foods lack fiber, nutrients, and enzymes. Processed foods come in bags, plastic, cans, and other containers.

These foods contain excessive sugars, coloring, dyes, dehydrogenated or partially dehydrogenated oils, MSG, flavor enhancers, preservatives, and many other unknown chemicals. They have been over baked, pasteurized, homogenized, cured, vacuum sealed, or killed in a hundred other ways.

These foods lack vitamins, minerals, nutrients, fiber, and life, which have been destroyed by heat, pressure, vacuum, and chemicals. Adding vitamins and minerals back into this food does not make it better, since manufacturers cannot duplicate nature. The vitamins and minerals added back into the food, are out of balance and do not have the right quantity.

Here are some of the foods to avoid:

- Alcohol, wine, and caffeine – they dehydrate the body by using up body fluids.

- Processed foods

- Coffee

- Dairy products – eggs, milk, cheese butter

- Margarine

- Fried foods

- Meat

- Raisin Bran

- Refined sugar
- Regular tea – Tea is rich in tannins, which are helpful for diarrhea, but interfere with colon peristaltic action.
- Salt
- Sodas
- Starch
- Sweets
- Cooked eggs, pasteurized milk, overcooked meat
- Mashed potatoes with gravy
- Overcooked carbohydrates

Coffee and Tea

Coffee and tea have a tightening effect – astringent – on your colon and this produces constipation. Drinking coffee on some occasion will have the opposite effect and promotes a bowel movement.

Coffee or tea is not a recommended drink, when you have constipation or when you are trying to prevent constipation. This is not true of most herbal teas, which do not contain caffeine.

The caffeine can be found in,

Ground percolated coffee, 8 oz. ------- 200 mg

Brewed tea, 8 oz. ---------------------- 75 mg

Soft drinks ----------------------------- 40 mg

Chocolate ----------------------------- 10 – 40 mg

Painkillers ---------------------------- 60 mg

Fried or Fatty Foods, Meats

Eating meat, bacon, sausage, and other fatty foods are constipating. These foods and others like butter, cheese, and eggs provide an excess of saturated fat and cholesterol that can easily stick to your colon walls. Cholesterol clings to your colon walls, just as it does in your arteries and organs.

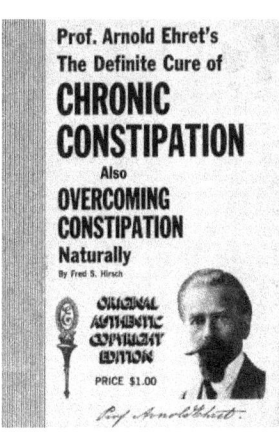

In his small booklet, Prof. Arnold Ehret's The Definite cure of Chronic Constipation, 1975, Fred S. Hirsch, quotes Prof Arnold Ehret who considers, "All fatty foods as being harmful and extremely constipating: clogging up the intestinal tract causing the entire system to become overloaded with their toxic waste. As we grow older the body's vital energy is depleted; through faulty diet, elimination is practically stop."

Meat

All kinds of meat are free fiber and this makes them constipating. Meat moves slower through your colon than other foods.

Since people eat a lot of meat at one sitting, undigested proteins make their way into your colon, which are fermented by bad bacteria. This decay creates a condition favorable for bad bacteria to multiply. When this happens, this is the start of many diseases that occur in your colon.

It is always best to eat plenty of uncooked vegetables, when eating meat. This provides fiber to help meat move quicker and safely through your colon.

Milk and Other Dairy Products

Dairy products are associated with constipation. This includes milk, cream soups, cheese, yogurt, some and desserts and baked goods.

The best dairy product to eat is cottage cheese. It is the least harmful to the body of all dairy products.

Eggs

Eggs, cheese, and butter are constipating and form toxic wastes, which poison your body.

Sodas

Soft drinks are high in phosphates. This chemical is used to dissolve sugar and to make soda taste better. When you drink soda, the phosphates combine with your calcium. If you do not have enough calcium in your blood or lymph liquid, phosphates pull it out of your bones.

Drinking sodas leads to lower levels of calcium in your body. You need calcium to help keep your colon clean.

Sweets

Most sweets are made from highly processed ingredients and an abundance of sugar. Because sweets are unnatural food and contain no fiber, they contribute directly to constipation and should be avoided.

Sugars in sweets and in all other types of foods have a deteriorating affect on your body. Sugars in your body break down into many chemicals, one, which is alcohol. If you drink soda, the sugar in the soda supplies the body and brain with the alcohol ethanol.

Eat more nutritious food

The foods listed below activate peristalsis and have plenty of fiber.

- apricots apples cantaloupe avocado

- figs blackberries kiwi strawberries

- grapes cherries dates peaches

- raspberries pears pineapples oranges

- nectarines coconuts mangos papayas

- Persimmons plums prunes raisins

- cranberries   elderberries   currants gooseberries

- bananas

- collard greens kale dark green lettuce

- mustard greens spinach chard cabbage

- dandelion greens endives corn brussels sprouts

- eggplants asparagus Jerusalem artichoke,

- rhubarb   rutabagas   carrots   celery cauliflower

- peas tomatoes turnips zucchini beets

- potatoes broccoli pumpkin corn squash
- bean sprouts green beans parsnip sweet potatoes
- radish peppers onions olives
- dulse chicory dandelion parsley watercress
- sesame seeds walnuts pumpkin seeds pecans
- peanuts black walnuts almonds flaxseed
- lentils soybeans beans broad beans black beans
- pinto beans kidney beans chickpeas lima beans baked beans
- navy beans
- millet oats barley whole grains spinach pasta
- whole wheat pasta

Minimize cooking of vegetable, since it reduces or breaks down the fiber.

Eat vegetables with skins when possible.

Broccoli has an anticancer compound called sulforaphane. This compound provides some protection against various types of cancer, when used with 750 mg of N-acetyl-cysteine, NAC. The reason you want to take NAC is that it provides glutathione that works with sulforaphane to fight cancer. Add this vegetable and supplement to your diet to prevent colon cancer.

Eat more fiber

If you are a cereal eater, this is a good time to eat more fiber. If not, then you can prepare a high fiber smoothie. Use more whole raw bran in your cereals. Or, you can grind up nuts and seed to add to your food.

Eating more fruits and vegetable will definitely give you more fiber.

Beans Stop Constipation

Beans are high in soluble and insoluble fiber. Eating them helps to prevent constipation and contributes to lowering your cholesterol. Beans become viscous, a thick heavy fluid, as they pass through the intestines. This viscous fiber fluid is of benefit in your colon, where it activates peristaltic action and promotes bowel movements.

Aside from lowering blood cholesterol and pressure, this viscous fiber in beans helps to decrease many types of colon diseases – cancer, colitis, and diverticulosis.

Most all types of beans have close to the same nutritional value. So eat the type you enjoy and gain its benefit.

One cup of cooked pinto or kidney beans has around 20 grams of fiber per cooked cup. Lima and White beans have around 16 grams of fiber.

Try not to eat beans from cans. You have no control in their preparation. It is best to cook your own beans in a crook pot by first,

- Rinsing beans to remove dirt, tiny rocks, and bad beans

- Soaking beans for 4-8 hours in water

- Dump the water from the soaked beans.

- Rinsing beans again but use distilled or reverse osmosis water

- Place beans into the crook pot and cover with distilled water or reverse osmosis water

- Add a couple of garlic cloves, onions, and your favorite chili powder.

- Turn crock-pot to low (not high) and cook beans for 8hours or until beans are soft.

You can turn your crock-pot on low when you go to bed, and in the morning, you will have cooked beans to eat for that day.

Health Alert: If you suffer from gout avoid beans, since they are high in purine.

Eat Good Oils

Good oil such as olive, flaxseed, evening primrose, black currant, and borage seed provide lubrication to the lining of your intestines and your colon. This lubrication is necessary for you to have regular bowel movements. Use these oils in place of mineral or castor oil.

Evening Primrose Oil - take 500 mg three times daily.

Omega-3 is found in flax seeds and in fish, such as Alaskan salmon, tilapia, rainbow trout, cod and halibut. It is an essential oil, this means that our body does not produce it and must be obtained from foods. Without omega-3 in your diet you will be prone to constipation, pain and many other diseases.

Fish

Do not eat fish for dinner. It is ok for lunch. Fish is hard to digest and you want to avoid foods that take too much time to digest, during the evening.

Fish Oil

Fish oil contains omega-3 fatty acids, which are essential for good health. It has the much needed fatty acids EPA, eicosapentaenoic acid and DHA, docosahexaenoic acid.

Fatty acids help reduce inflammation through prostaglandin production. Prostaglandin's help reduces inflammation in your colon, which helps make your colon work better and reduces the possibility of constipation.

Health Tip: Use the enteric-coated fish oil capsules to reduce colon inflammation and to help reduce constipation.

Health Alert: Make sure when taking fish oil that is it is not fish liver oil. They are not the same food product.

Health Drug Alert: Fish oil can increase the rate of bleeding, if you are using anticoagulant drugs such as warfarin, coumadin, or platelet inhibiting drugs - aspirin or ticlopidine.

Recommend dose of fish oil is 1000 to 1500 mg each day.

Flax Seeds

Flax seeds and its oil fall in the top 10 of healthy foods to live on. It contains a high-level of omega-3 fatty acids that are essential for life. You cannot live without the omega-3 fatty acids. Your diet must consist of a 3:1 or 4:1 ratio of omega-6 to omega 3. You must have 3 or 4 parts of omega-6 to 1 part of omega-3 in your diet. Unfortunately, this is hard to measure, so just make sure you are using flax seed oil and supplementing with fish oil in your diet.

Without this balance and with too much omega-6 fatty acid in your diet you will be prone to illnesses related to,

- Autoimmune diseases

- Breast cancer

- Cardiovascular diseases

- Excessive blood clotting

- Over drive of the immune system

Aside from all the benefits flax seeds provide, it contains the fiber and oils that will help prevent constipation. It contains 66% insoluble and 33% soluble fiber. Here is the nutritional breakdown for flax seeds.

- Fat 41% - 57% is omega 3, 18% monounsaturated, 16% omega-6, 9% saturated
- Fiber 28%
- Protein 20%
- Moisture 7%
- Ash 4%

The 57% omega-3 is considered plant source and differs from the omega-3 found in fish. Flax seed omega-3 is considered short chain fatty acid and fish omega-3 is long chain fatty acid.

Your body only converts a small amount of flax seed omega-3 oil to EPA, fish long chain fatty acid. Because of this, you may want to also add fish oil to your diet, if you want the benefits of a higher level of EPA.

The recommendation for getting the proper amount of omega-3 into your diet is to eat fish 4 times a week and 1 ½ teaspoon of flax seeds. Not many people meet this requirement.

So here is what you can do to get more omega-

3 in your diet, so you can offset the bad affects too much omega-6 and reduce and prevent constipation. Use 1-3 tablespoon of flax seed daily. Always grind these seeds with a coffee grinder. Then add them to your food.

- Add 1 teaspoon to your smoothie

- Add 1 teaspoon to your salad dressing

- Add 1 teaspoon to your cereal

Health tip: Use flax seed without heating them. This preserves the nutritive value of this food and prevents its oxidation, which produces free radicals that are not good for your health.

Garlic

Include raw garlic in your diet and cooking. Garlic destroys harmful bacteria in your colon and penetrates your colon walls to loosen up accumulated waste.

Also, you can use aged garlic extract, which comes in a capsule. Aged garlic promotes the growth of good bacteria in your colon. Also aged garlic absorbs heavy metals from your blood. Heavy metals are responsible for cell degradation.

Health tip: Avoid using powdered garlic, since all its nutritive value has been lost, during its heating process.

Lecithin for Nerve protection

Lecithin is needed to build the protective layer that surrounds your nerves that network throughout your body. Without this protective layer or with a worn layer, the information that is transmitted along the nerves suffers interference. This interference distorts the information that is sent from your brain to your body, causing diseases.

The nerve network that surrounds your colon needs to be strong and stable, since it is constantly reacting to peristaltic activity.

Lecithin can be purchased in granules. You can use it as an additive to many of your food preparations – smoothies, cereal, soups, salads, sauces, and gravies. This is easy to do since it adds no flavor to your food.

Lecithin consists of 10-15% choline. Choline is used by the body to form acetylcholine. Acetylcholine is a neuro- transmitter that is active in recalling memories.

Lecithin is one supplement that you must add to your eating pattern. It helps to break up fat to tiny bubbles that prevent it from sticking to your artery walls.

Exercise

Exercise is necessary for reducing or minimizing constipation. By exercising, you can promote, produce, or create the following:

- Tones and strengthen your colon muscles

- Eliminates blood toxins by sweating.

- Stimulates your cells to eliminate waste and have

- stimulates your lymphatic system to eliminate waste

- Reduces tension and anxiety

- Stimulates your colons wall cell structure to increase its metabolic rate and thus improve its function.

Daily walks, after a meal, stimulate your colon for bowel movements. In addition, walking strengthens and tones your colon walls. This prevents your colon from becoming misshaped, when you on occasion become constipated.

Health Tip: Inactivity or lack of exercise will contribute to lack of colon muscle tone, which will contribute to constipation no matter what your age.

There are many good exercises that stimulate and strengthen your body. Any type of exercise will be of benefit to your health. When your colon is toxic, then exercises that activate the lymph system are good.

The lymph system removes waste and toxins from the liquid that surround your cells. So it is critical these toxins not be allowed to remain in your body long. If they do, then this is another form of constipation. Lymph nodes get plugged up with toxins, waste, and bacteria and as more waste and toxins are created they get backed up in the lymph liquid or vessels.

The rebounder has long been known to be one of the best exercise tools for stimulating and activating the lymphatic system. It also strengthens all the internal organs, tissues and cells.

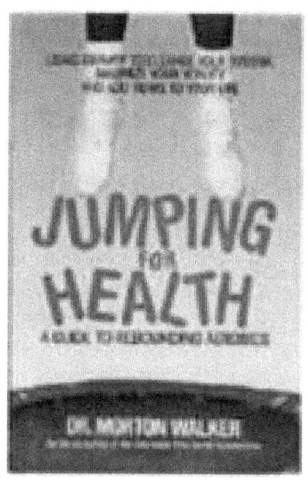

In, Jumping for Health, 1989, Dr. Morton Walker, identifies why the re-bounder is good for a healthy body, "Thus, the G force at the top of the bounce is eliminated and the body becomes weightless for a fraction of a second. At the bottom of the bounce when you touch the mat the G force suddenly doubles over what is ordinary gravity on earth and internal organs are put under pressure. Their cellular stimulation is increased accordingly so waste materials within cells get squeezed out. The lymphatic system carries waste away to be disposed of through the urinary and other excretory mechanisms. Rebounding makes the body cleaner."

Dr. Morton continues,

"The increased G force also puts cell walls under stress causing them to undergo an individual training effect. The aerobics of rebounding brings more oxygen for penetration by osmosis from the blood. Each cell gets the amount of nourishment it requires on which to thrive."

And Finally,

"This combination of excretion of wastes and incorporation of nourishment, both done more efficiently than any ordinary program of exercise, conditions the cells beyond their usual threshold. They get stronger and gain endurance to cope better with the stresses encountered in daily life Because of your habits you have created the body you have now. If you are happy with your body and are in good health, then you may not need to make many changes or any changes at all."

But, if you are not satisfied with your body, the illnesses you support and the thoughts you think and carry with you, then look at some of the changes you can make that will make your life happier and healthier.

Daily Walks

Walking is an essential exercise to prevent constipation. It must be done every day and the best time is early morning. Walking is the right movement to stimulate your bowel so constipation is avoided.

Try to walk briskly for ½ hour and consistency is the key. Try to keep to a regular program of exercise.

Other types of exercise are also good. The main thing is to provide movement for your stomach area. This provides movement to your colon and helps to move fecal matter through your colon. It strengthens your colon walls and helps to release glutamine that feeds the intestinal cell lining.

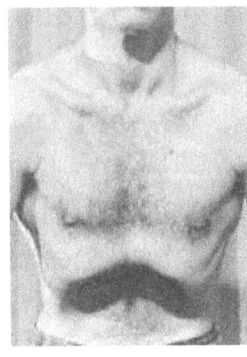 In 1963, Richard L. Hittleman, in his book called, Be Young With Yoga, described an exercise called the "Abdominal Lift." This is another exercise that can be done to strengthen your colon. The benefits of this exercise are:

- Gives your colon, intestines, kidneys, liver, pancreas and stomach stimulation that brings in blood to carry away toxins.

- Stimulates peristaltic action, which helps to relieve and prevent constipation

Here's how to do it.

In a standing position with knee slightly bent and hands on upper thighs, draw in stomach area and push air out of your mouth. Hold this position for a moment as shown in photo then snap stomach out.

Then without breathing, continue to bring stomach in and immediately snapping it out Do this 3-4 times before breathing. Do this exercise for 5 breaths.

Feed the Good Bacteria

The good bacteria, in your colon, are known by many names – good bacteria, micro flora, and probiotics. These bacteria are necessary for good colon and body health. The main bacteria in your colon are:

- Lactobacillus acidophilus
- Bifidobacterium bifidum
- Lactobacillus salivarius
- Bifidobacterium infantis
- Streptococcus faecium

When buying probiotics, you should buy a mixture of these bacteria. In some products you will find added **Fructo-oligosccharides**, **FOS**, which helps feed the good bacteria and promote their survival.

Cultured yogurt is a good way to get additional good bacteria into your colon. The best way to eat it is in-between meals. The best yogurt to eat is goat milk yogurt. It costs a bit more, but it is worth the health benefits you get from it.

Look for yogurt that says the bacteria culture was added after pasteurization. If the yogurt was pasteurized after the bacteria culture was added, the good bacteria have been destroyed.

Eat yogurt at least 3 times a week. You can add flax seed oil, berries, raisins, flax seed grounds, or other toppings that promotes bowel movements.

The best way to get good bacteria into your colon is to take a probiotic supplement, liquid or pill, between meals with distilled water. When probiotics are taken with food, your stomach acid will destroy the probiotic benefit.

Eating cultured vegetables is another way to get probiotics or good bacteria. Some flora-enhanced foods are:

- Sauerkraut

- Yogurt

- Kefir

- Miso

- Micro alga

Taking a Good Mineral Supplement

To maintain a strong and active colon, you need to take a good mineral supplement, which contains plenty of sodium, magnesium, calcium, and potassium. In addition, you need to get these minerals from the food you eat. Food has a balance of these minerals and nutrient that you need to build your colon and other parts of your body.

Potassium

Potassium is needed to keep your colon walls working properly and for keeping them free of acid, which attracts disease. It helps to dislodge colon wastes that accumulate along your colon walls.

Potassium tastes bitter, so most bitter foods contain potassium, especially herbal teas. Best foods to eat for high levels of potassium are:

Cucumbers	apples
Bitter greens	lentils
apple cider vinegar	
American prunes	
Almonds	bananas
Oatmeal	beans
Potato skins	blueberries
German prunes	goat milk
grapes	apricots
Peaches	pears
Gooseberries	raisins
Romaine lettuce	tomatoes
Figs	sesame seeds
Carrots	beets and prunes

Prepare a Miracle Mineral Salad

Cut up romaine or dark green lettuce, Chopped garlic cloves, onions, 2-3 tablespoons of apple cider vinegar, and add hard-boiled eggs

The allicin in the garlic is invigorated by the minerals in the onion, causing the allicin to penetrate the large intestine wall. The fiber, in green vegetables, helps to scrub the intestinal walls. The apple vinegar boosts enzymatic action of the allicin and the allicin stimulates the peristaltic movement. This is a natural way to dissolve accumulated toxic wastes on your colon wall.

To make this salad more potent, make a salad dressing by combining.

- juice to two cloves of garlic

- 2 tablespoon of flaxseed oil

- 3 tablespoons of olive oil

- 1 tablespoon of balsamic vinegar

- 2 tablespoons of apple cider vinegar

- ground up flax seeds, sunflower see

- one tablespoon of bran

Digestive enzymes

Digestive enzymes help you digest and absorb your food and supplements. Your body produces different enzymes to digest different types of food such as,

- Protease – for digesting protein

- Lactase – for digesting lactose a protein in milk

- Amylase – for digesting carbohydrate

- Pepsin – for digesting protein

Medical Alert: Do not use digestive enzymes, if you have problems with ulcers.

Amylase starts carbohydrate digestion in your mouth. The longer you chew your food, which is a healthy practice, the better digested your food will be. Your stomach will not have to work as hard and less undigested food will reach your colon.

Fruits and vegetables have their own digestive enzymes, which help your stomach to digest them. When fruits or vegetables are heated above 120 F, their enzymes are destroyed and no longer available for your body. When this happens, your body has to create these enzymes to digest this cooked food. This takes energy and enzymes away from within your body that could be used elsewhere to do more important work.

When you eat cooked food and processed and packaged foods, you use excessive digestive enzymes. Sometimes not all your food is digested properly, and these undigested remains move into your colon where they create gas, toxic material, which weakens your colon wall.

18: How to Stop Constipation

Where to Start

I have given you plenty of information on how to relieve your constipation and how to prevent it. Just by applying many of these health ideas and tips, you are well on your way to creating excellent health and, of course, relieving your constipation.

I know that some of you will be confused about what to do first or where to start.

Each one of you will start by using different remedies. The ones you choose would depend on what you are familiar with, what you like to eat, what you have on hand, or how severe you are constipated.

Constipation Program

A program to help you have regular bowel movements and to help you prevent having constipation consists of some basic steps. From the information and remedies discussed in the previous chapters, you can experiment and test different ones and use the ones that work best for you.

In the case where you have had long-term constipation, it may be necessary to retrain your colon to have bowel movements. If this is the case, you may have to consult your doctor or an alternative medicine practitioner to get their direction.

Constipation Steps

To get relief from frequent or occasionally constipation, these are the steps and changes you need to consider.

Chose a natural laxative to relieve your constipation

- Eliminate constipating habits

- Improve your digestion

- Improve your diet

- Keep your good bacteria dominant in your colon

- Make your colon acidic

- Retrain your bowels for regularity

- Strengthen colon and surrounding areas

- Choose a natural laxative to relieve you constipation

Which natural laxative should you choose? I would recommend you choose 3 different ways to start relieving your constipation and use them at the same time.

First, I would recommend using Tripahal. Use it as directed on the bottle.

Second, start adding more fiber to your diet. If you eat oats or multigrain cream cereal, add bran to it. Or grind up some flax seed, sunflower seeds, sesame seeds or almonds and add it to your cereal. Make sure you drink more water during the day, if you do this.

Third, add a juice or vegetable remedy you like and use it every day for a week or so. Eat more fruits daily between meals and at other free times.

One of method to use is to take 2 capsules of each cayenne pepper and MSM after each meal. Also drink apple juice, and eat 2 apples each day, eat other fruits, eat oats, and various seeds. And of course, eat fresh vegetables every day. There are other foods that you can eat and those are listed in the chapters you have just read.

Eliminate Constipating Habits

Look at what constipating habits you have. Start changing them one by one. For example, on the first week you could concentrate on drinking more water. Start taking a quart of water to work in a glass jar. Add a small amount lemon to it to give a little flavor.

During the following week concentrate on eating more fruits and vegetables. Start taking apples to work or strips of carrots, celery, or other vegetables you like for snacks.

On the third week, you could concentrate on making and eating an evening salad every day of that week, if you are not already doing this.

On the fourth week, start adding more fiber to your diet.

Look at some of the other areas you need to change.

- Stop using Drugstore laxatives

- Start exercising more

- Drink more water

- Start going to the rest room when you have the urge for a bowel movement

These are the constipating habits you need to change. Start changing these habits one by one. Each day look at the list of good and bad habits to change and increase or decrease the habit as necessary.

Improve your digestion

By improving your digestion, you stop undigested food from reaching your colon, where it can become putrefied.

You can help your digestion and improve your body's health by taking digestive enzymes at each meal. Taking digestive enzymes is almost a must for the elderly. They typically lack HCL acid to digest protein and need to take an HCL- pepsin supplement. And it would not hurt to take a regular enzyme supplement with it.

Improve your diet

There is no doubt you need to change your diet. Constipation is caused by not eating the right foods and eating foods that are constipating.

Fiber

Eating food with plenty of fiber is a requirement. There are many fruits and vegetables with plenty of fiber. You need to eat those foods that have plenty of soluble and non-soluble fiber. Eating only fruits and vegetable that contain mainly soluble fiber will not help you prevent or to stop constipation.

You also need those foods with plenty of non-soluble fiber, which add bulk, draw water, and add density to your stools. This type of fiber helps your fecal matter to move through your colon easier and quicker.

Bran

Bran is helpful in providing non-soluble fiber. It is better to use plain bran rather than cereals with added bran. But in case you cannot find raw bran, then a second choice is a cereal that contains processed bran and is high in fiber. Use this second choice bran, only until your constipation is cleared.

It is better to use rice, oat, or corn bran rather than wheat bran. Mix the bran in your morning cereal – rolled oats, multigrain cereal - pancakes, smoothies, salads, and wherever you feel it will taste good.

How much fiber should you eat? Eat between 30 – 40 mg of fiber every day. Fiber is one of the keys to keeping free of constipation.

If you are doing all the right things for improving the flow of fecal matter through your colon, and you still have constipation, then you need to see your doctor. This might be a sign of some underlying illness, where you need a doctor's help.

Good Bacteria

Keeping your good bacteria dominant in your colon can be difficult, if you have become unbalance with excessive bad bacteria. The first step you need to take is to start feeding your good bacteria. You can do this by using edible dairy whey or FOS. You should also start eating those foods that feed your good bacteria.

In cases, where you have used medical drugs for a long time, drink alcohol, use drugstore laxatives, or have been constipated for some time, you may have to resort to implanting good bacteria into your colon using an enema.

The technique for this has been discussed in Dave Webster's book, Acidophilus and Colon Health. It is something not covered in this book.

Make your colon acidic

Making and keeping your colon acidic, requires you eat the right kind of food, have good digestion, and have a good mental attitude. The foods you should be eating are listed in the previous chapters. When you eat processed foods with little fiber and excess food additives, this changes your colon from acidic to an alkaline and helps the bad bacteria to multiple.

Keeping a negative attitude and having anxiety, also affects your colon. A continual tightening of your colon walls overworks your colon and eventually weakens it. A weaken colon is more susceptible to constipation, which favors the growth of bad bacteria.

Retrain your bowels for regularity

Long-term constipation can come from your colon's inability to create peristaltic movement. This can result from long-term use of laxatives, use of pharmaceutical drugs, ignoring the signal to have a bowel movement, eating excessive process food, lack of fiber in your diet, and having excessive tension in your life.

To retrain your colon to have regular bowel movements, start by,

- Take 4000 to 5000 mg of MSM torpedoes
- Eating your meals at the same time every day
- Sit down on the toilet at the same time every morning and midday
- Use a herbal combination laxative that will gentle stimulate peristaltic action
- Consider learn some relaxation techniques to lessen any anxiety or tension you may be experiencing
- Follow the list of other actions to take to reduce constipation in this chapter.
- Use natural laxatives to help retrain and strengthen bowels
- Strengthen colon and surrounding areas

How do you strengthen your colon? Getting the proper amount of minerals, vitamins, and oils into your body does this. Minerals help to build body cells and tissue. Use a mineral supplement like Alkalife or any other electrolyte type liquid mineral. Get your oils by using olive and flax oil in your salads and soups.

Exercise

No exercise is an unhealthy practice. Body movement in the abdominal area is necessary for good colon health. This movement comes from exercise such as running, walking, sit-ups, massage, and yoga stomach movements.

Exercise helps to tone and build colon wall tissue and muscle. It helps in moving fecal matter through your colon, since exercise stretches and contracts your colon similar to what happens during peristaltic action.

A great exercise is rebounding. This is one of the best exercises, since it helps tone your whole body and activate your lymphatic system, so your body fluid moves easily.

There is also another great exercise program called PACE. This program is one of the better exercise programs available, since you don't have to spend hours exercising. You do quick and fast exercises to get your heart rate up. With this program, your exercise time can be reduced to half an hour or so.

Final Comments

As you change your diet, especially if you add more juices, fruits, and vegetables, you are going to experience cleansing of your body. What this means is you will experience some discomfort or slight pain throughout your body as toxins are released and look for a way out of your body. As toxins come out of your cells and organs their acidity causes pain. Your body's minerals will neutralize some of this acid. That is why it is important to use a mineral supplement and to eat plenty of fruits and vegetables.

You may experience more mucus discharge as these toxins work their way out of your elimination ports. You may experience more mucus coming out of your nose, throat, and mouth. Mucus will also find its way into your colon and out the rectum in stools.

During this cleansing period, do not take any medication to stop or eliminate nasal drainage. You may also develop rashes or other skin eruptions as toxins come out through your skin.

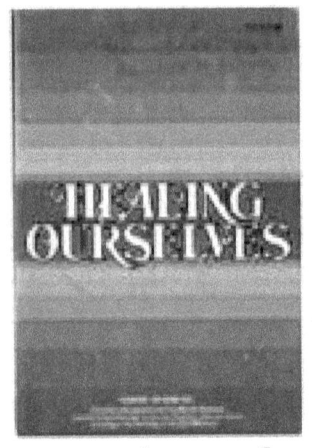

In his book, Healing Ourselves, 1973, Nabors Marmot from his studies of oriental medicine for thirty year, talks about the cleansing process. "A discharge can last one week, sometimes two, and in some cases even longer. The strength and duration of the discharge depends generally on past eating habits and the method of cure being employed. The use of compresses or herbs will hasten the discharge."

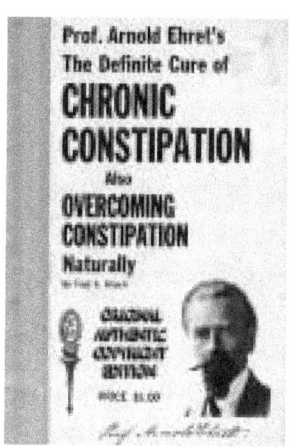

I complete this e-book with the words of Fred S. Hirsch who wrote in 1975, in his small green booklet, "Constipation is a clogging-up of the entire human pipe-system. Nature wisely stores the undigested, toxic wastes 'temporarily' in the tissues, awaiting an early opportunity to dispose of these poisons! Sickness is such an opportunity – 'acute disease' is Nature's attempt to eliminate the stored-up 'sewage' and the 'healing Process' differs according to the physical condition of each individual"

19: About the Author

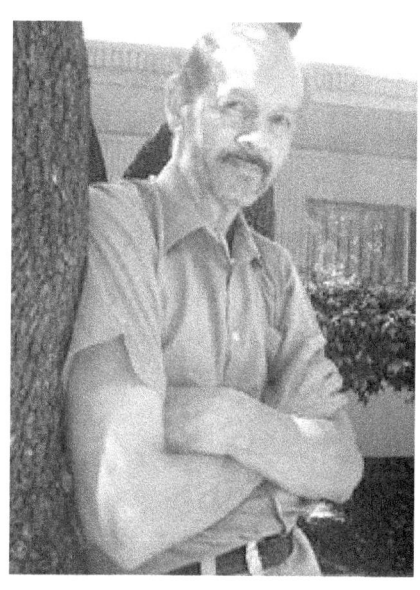

Thank you for taking time to read my e-book. I sincerely hope that there are some remedies and procedures here that will help give you relief and hopefully a cure for your constipation. Here are some additional e-books that I have written that will also help you gain better health.

Rudy Silva is a natural nutritional consultant educated in the United States in Nutrition and Physics. He is a graduate from the

University of San Jose State in California. He is author of 45 other e-books on natural remedies. He has authored a newsletter in natural remedies for over 4 years.

He is now living in the Philippines where he writes nutrition and remedy e-books. He is also helping many clients reach new levels of health.

Resource pages

Here is other kindle e-book about using natural remedies that have been written by this author. You can see the entire list at:

http://tinyurl.com/b2f7wd3

Acne Remedies
Natural Help With Acne
Best natural acne treatments: Acne facial
Constipation Remedies
The Best Constipation Remedies
Best Constipated Women Natural Cures
How to Relieve Constipation with Fruits
Essential Fatty Acids
Taking The Mystery Out Of Essential Fatty acids
Amazing Fish Oil Benefits Revealed
Nutrition Remedies

Updated Version - Secret Diet And Nutrition
Secret Healthy Fruit Practices Revealed
Fast Healing Juice Nutrition Therapy: Nutrition Tips 3
Fantastic Alkaline Fruit Benefits Revealed
Calcium (Discover How To Use Calcium To Avoid Devastating Diseases)
Stomach Remedies
Acid Reflux: Fast and Easy Cures For Acid Reflux
Asthma Treatment Cures With Remedies
How To Do Natural Colon Cleansing
Gastrointestinal Digestion Secrets Revealed
Misc. Remedies
Natural Hair Loss Treatment: Women And Men
Effective Natural Hemorrhoids Treatment
Iron Deficiency Anemia
Secrets To Understanding Behavior
Fast Acting Ear Infection Remedies

If you need support or want to promote any of his e-books, please contact him at rss41@yahoo.com. He looks forward to hearing from you.

Checkout all his other books at:

http://tinyurl.com/b2f7wd3

Give A Review

And, don't forget to give a review for this e-book at Amazon so that others can gain the benefits of what is in this e-book. Just write a few sentences and that is sufficient.

To you, for creating better health and more happiness in your life,

Rudy S Silva

www.ingramcontent.com/pod-product-compliance
Lightning Source LLC
Chambersburg PA
CBHW070847290526
45795CB00001B/16